The Sociology of Medical Screening

Sociology of Health and Illness Monograph Series

Edited by Hannah Bradby
School of Health and Human Sciences
University of Essex
Wivenhoe Park
Colchester C04 3SQ
UK

Current titles

The Sociology of Medical Screening
Critical Perspectives, New Directions

Edited by

Natalie Armstrong and Helen Eborall

⟨Ⓦ⟩WILEY-BLACKWELL

A John Wiley & Sons, Ltd., Publication

This edition first published 2012
Originally published as Volume 34, Issue 2 of *The Sociology of Health & Illness*
Chapters © 2012 The Authors.
Book Compilation © 2012 Foundation for the Sociology of Health & Illness/Blackwell Publishing Ltd.

Blackwell Publishing was acquired by John Wiley & Sons in February 2007. Blackwell's publishing program has been merged with Wiley's global Scientific, Technical, and Medical business to form Wiley-Blackwell.

Registered Office
John Wiley & Sons Ltd, The Atrium, Southern Gate, Chichester, West Sussex, PO19 8SQ, United Kingdom

Editorial Offices
350 Main Street, Malden, MA 02148-5020, USA
9600 Garsington Road, Oxford, OX4 2DQ, UK
The Atrium, Southern Gate, Chichester, West Sussex, PO19 8SQ, UK

For details of our global editorial offices, for customer services, and for information about how to apply for permission to reuse the copyright material in this book please see our website at www.wiley.com/wiley-blackwell.

The rights of Natalie Armstrong and Helen Eborall to be identified as the authors of the editorial material in this work has been asserted in accordance with the UK Copyright, Designs and Patents Act 1988.

Wiley also publishes its books in a variety of electronic formats. Some content that appears in print may not be available in electronic books.

Designations used by companies to distinguish their products are often claimed as trademarks. All brand names and product names used in this book are trade names, service marks, trademarks or registered trademarks of their respective owners. The publisher is not associated with any product or vendor mentioned in this book. This publication is designed to provide accurate and authoritative information in regard to the subject matter covered. It is sold on the understanding that the publisher is not engaged in rendering professional services. If professional advice or other expert assistance is required, the services of a competent professional should be sought.

Library of Congress Cataloging-in-Publication Data

The sociology of medical screening: critical perspectives, new directions / edited by Natalie Armstrong and Helen Eborall.
       p. cm.
   "Originally published as Volume 34, Issue 2 of The Sociology of Health & Illness".
   Includes index.
     ISBN 978-1-118-23178-4 (pbk.)
   I. Armstrong, Natalie.   II. Eborall, Helen.   III. Sociology of health & illness.
   [DNLM: 1. Mass Screening.   2. Genetic Testing.   3. Sociology, Medical.   WA 245]

   362.196′04207–dc23

                                        2012009305

A catalogue record for this book is available from the British Library.

Cover design by Design Deluxe.

Set in 9.5/11.5 pt Times NR Monotype by Toppan Best-set Premedia Limited
Printed in Malaysia by Ho Printing (M) Sdn Bhd

1   2012

Contents

Notes on Contributors

David Armstrong   Department of Primary Care and Public Health Sciences, King's College London.

Natalie Armstrong   Department of Health Sciences, University of Leicester.

Mara Buchbinder   Department of Social Medicine, University of North Carolina, Chapel Hill, North Carolina, USA.

Helen Eborall   Department of Health Sciences, University of Leicester.

Alex Faulkner   Department of Political Economy, King's College London.

Chris Gillespie   Department of Sociology, Brandeis University, Waltham, Massachusetts, USA.

Stuart Hogarth   Department of Social Science, Health and Medicine, King's College London.

Michael Hopkins   SPRU – Science and Technology Policy Research, University of Sussex.

Janina Kehr   Medizinhistorisches Institut und Museum, Universität Zürich, Zürich, Switzerland.

Lene Koch   Steno Health Promotion Centre, Gentofte, Denmark.

Alison Pilnick   School of Sociology and Social Policy, University of Nottingham.

Julie Roberts   Warwick Medical School, University of Warwick.

Victor Rodriguez   Department of Legal and Economic Governance Studies, University of Twente.

Nete Schwennesen   Steno Health Promotion Centre, Gentofte, Denmark.

Stefan Timmermans   Department of Sociology, UCLA, Los Angeles, California, USA.

Olga Zayts   Department of Linguistics, University of Hong Kong.

1

The sociology of medical screening: past, present and future

Natalie Armstrong and Helen Eborall

Introduction

Screening for medical conditions is an important and topical issue. The potential reach of population-based medical screening is growing and developing; it is now possible to screen for an increasing number of conditions, using ever-more advanced and sophisticated technologies. Medical screening, a key strategy of preventive medicine, raises fundamental issues for sociological inquiry because screening is a social intervention as well as a medical one, and can raise important social dilemmas. At present, however, a well-developed sociology of medical screening is lacking.

As we will go on to explore in more detail below, we believe that sociological work on screening is currently fragmented and has yet to constitute more than the sum of its individual parts. We suggest a number of factors might be contributing to this. First, sociological work on screening tends to be located in a wide range of sub-disciplines without a great deal of cross-fertilisation between and across these. Secondly, much of this work tends to be confined to studies of screening for particular conditions, and hence may remain largely contained within specialist silos. Thirdly, we would suggest that sociological work on screening currently remains somewhat limited in its analytical scope.

This collection has three main aims. First, through both this introduction and David Armstrong's contribution, we seek to reflect on both the nature of screening itself and the sociological attention it has received to date in order to provide an introduction for those new to this area. Secondly, we reflect on sociology's potential contribution to wider debates about screening, and propose future research directions. Thirdly, we showcase a range of work that constitutes the sociology of screening as it currently stands. This collection of new essays addresses a range of issues from a variety of theoretical and methodological approaches. Taken together, they demonstrate current sociological concerns around screening, and make clear suggestions for how research in this area should develop in the future. Our ultimate wish is that this collection should serve to stimulate and inspire future research on medical screening that starts to achieve the cross-fertilisation of ideas and the production of theoretical approaches that may have purchase across the area of screening as a whole. Before we can embark on those tasks, though, we begin by explaining what we mean by screening, and why we believe screening merits and, indeed, requires sociological attention.

The Sociology of Medical Screening, First Edition. Edited by Natalie Armstrong and Helen Eborall. Chapters © 2012 The Authors. Book Compilation © 2012 Foundation for the Sociology of Health & Illness / Blackwell Publishing Ltd. Published 2012 by Blackwell Publishing Ltd.

What do we mean by screening?

The focus of this collection of essays is population-based medical screening; by which we mean screening offered to all people within an identified target population; for example, based on age and/or sex. This is fundamentally different from both the traditional medical model of diagnosis following a patient's spontaneous presentation of symptoms, and opportunistic case finding in which a doctor tests for a condition during a consultation about another matter. Rather, it involves the purposeful application of tests to an asymptomatic population in order to classify people into those who are *unlikely* to have or develop a disease and those who are *likely* to have or develop a disease. In the UK, the National Screening Committee (UKNSC) assesses the evidence for screening programmes and advises the government about implementation (National Screening Committee 2011). The UKNSC defines screening as:

> a process of identifying apparently healthy people who may be at increased risk
> of a disease or condition. They can then be offered information, further tests and
> appropriate treatment to reduce their risk and/or any complications arising from the
> disease or condition.

While misdiagnosis is of course possible, this crucial distinction from diagnosis means that all screening programmes involve an inescapable risk of false-positives and false-negatives, in which people are either incorrectly identified as at risk (and therefore subjected to unnecessary further investigation and possibly treatment) or are falsely reassured (and therefore not offered the further investigation and treatment they may require). The distinction from diagnosis is also important from a sociological position; the sociology of screening should not be confused with the sociology of diagnosis (Jutel and Nettleton 2011).

Globally, healthcare organisations differ with regard to the range of screening programmes offered, the groups targeted, the frequency of invitation, and the cost to the 'consumer' (which is obviously dependent on the country's system of healthcare provision). Costs aside, however, a similar position is taken by many developed countries in terms of currently available and recommended screening programmes. A full account of screening provision across these countries is beyond the scope of this essay. England is a useful example, however. Its current screening programmes include those for: cervical cancer; breast cancer; bowel/colorectal cancer; abdominal aortic aneurism; diabetic retinopathy; and a range of antenatal and newborn screening (including fetal anomalies, infectious diseases in pregnancy, newborn screening, newborn hearing screening, Sickle Cell and Thalassaemia, and the Newborn and Infant Physical Examination Programme). These programmes are systematic population screening programmes, meaning that the whole population eligible to be screened is invited to participate automatically – for example, upon reaching a set age – without having to indicate any prior interest. In contrast, further programmes that are in operation, but are not National Screening Committee approved systematic population screening programmes, include: a risk management programme for prostate cancer; Chlamydia screening; and the NHS health checks programme to assess risk of heart disease, type 2 diabetes, stroke and chronic kidney disease (Department of Health 2009). In addition to NHS provision, there has also been a marked increase in screening offered by private companies over recent years. Concerns that individuals could pay private companies for screening that might cause unnecessary anxiety and could lead to further unnecessary investigations have led the UK National Screening Committee to issue guidance on the pros and cons of private provision to both GPs and the public (Cole 2010).

Screening is costly. The cost of the breast cancer screening programme in England, for example, is now estimated at approximately £96 million per year (NHS Cancer Screening Programmes 2011a) and cervical screening (including the cost of treating cervical abnormalities) has been estimated to cost around £157 million a year in England (NHS Cancer Screening Programmes 2011b). To maximise cost effectiveness and efficiency, population-based screening programmes target the group(s) of people considered to be most at risk of developing or having a condition in relation to factors such as their age, sex, ethnicity, or physical attributes. Yet the cost effectiveness of a screening programme is by no means the only criterion assessed when considering implementation. Indeed, based on the underlying principle that screening must not do more harm than good, and in order to assure quality in the screening programmes implemented, the UK National Screening Committee requires that criteria about the condition, test, treatment and programme are all met before a programme is implemented (National Screening Committee 2011)[1]. These criteria still draw to a large extent on Wilson and Jungner's (1968) classic principles, as outlined in Box 1.

A note on genetic screening
Developments in technology now allow genetic screening for certain conditions and, in some cases, this is delivered through population-based screening. The most widespread example is the incorporation of genetic testing into newborn screening. In the UK this takes place via a heel prick to collect blood from the baby, and includes testing for phenylketonuria, congenital hypothyroidism, sickle cell disorders, cystic fibrosis and medium-chain acyl-CoA dehydrogenase deficiency or MCADD, and in the US includes over 50 conditions (Watson *et al.* 2006).

Predictive genetic testing is, of course, available for many other conditions (for example, Huntington's disease and hereditary breast and ovarian cancer) and has received notable sociological attention. Areas of study include the social and cultural impact of providing people with information relating to their risk for future disease (Davison *et al.* 1994, Cox and McKellin 1999); the experiences of genetic responsibility that testing and receiving the results may invoke (Hallowell 1999, Raspberry and Skinner 2011, Polzer *et al.* 2002); and how such genetic responsibility may be gendered (Steinberg 1996, Hallowell *et al.* 2006, Reed 2009). However, because genetic testing of this kind is not routinely offered, we believe it therefore cannot be considered as *population* screening; rather, individuals are referred

---

Box 1 *Wilson and Jungner's principles of screening (1968)*

(1) The condition sought should be an important health problem.
(2) There should be an accepted treatment for patients with recognised disease.
(3) Facilities for diagnosis and treatment should be available.
(4) There should be a recognisable latent or early symptomatic stage.
(5) There should be a suitable test or examination.
(6) The test should be acceptable to the population.
(7) The natural history of the condition, including development from latent to declared disease, should be adequately understood.
(8) There should be an agreed policy on whom to treat as patients.
(9) The cost of case-finding (including diagnosis and treatment of patients diagnosed) should be economically balanced in relation to possible expenditure on medical care as a whole.
(10) Case-finding should be a continuing process and not a 'once and for all' project.

for genetic testing by their doctor if there is a family history of a particular genetic condition/disorder or some types of cancer.

Why does screening merit sociological attention?

Screening programmes are social interventions as much as they are medical interventions, and they can pose challenging ethical, legal and social dilemmas, the sociological scrutiny of which can be particularly useful both in informing the policy, in development and implementation of screening programmes, but also in developing sociological theory. Debates and controversies about medical screening are rarely confined to policy makers and health professionals. Contestations about the science underlying population screening are common, and frequently enter the public sphere, engaging with wider societal themes and normative questions. For example, despite evidence that PSA testing does not reduce prostate cancer mortality and can instead cause harm from unnecessary treatment and anxiety, in the US a powerful pro-PSA lobby group contests this and encourages widespread screening. This position has been argued to be associated with the money to be gained by this group from men undergoing testing (Yamey and Wilkes 2002). Another example is the information leaflet on the UK Breast Screening Programme which was recently strongly criticised for being misleading, manipulative and not providing the basis for informed consent, as the harms (including over-diagnosis and over-treatment) were not clearly explained (Baum *et al.* 2009, Mayor 2010) in light of the growing evidence of the uncertainties and extent of over-diagnosis (Gøtzsche and Nielsen 2009, McPherson 2010).

The difficulty of establishing a screening test with maximum sensitivity and specificity (thereby avoiding as many false negative and false positive results as possible) is often underestimated and underrepresented in the popular press. Instead, pleas for new or extended screening programmes from lobby groups, which may be constructed as rights or entitlements, can overshadow the science – as demonstrated in the UK in 2009 when calls to reduce the age at which routine cervical screening commences were provoked by the high profile death of the reality television star Jade Goody at the age of 27. In 2003, the NHS Cervical Screening Programme in England had standardised the age at which women are first invited for cervical screening to 25 years (rather than the previous 20 years) and Jade Goody's death led to considerable pressure for a re-lowering of the starting age. This pressure endured even after the government's Advisory Committee on Cervical Screening reviewed this decision in May 2009 and agreed unanimously there should be no change (Advisory Committee on Cervical Screening 2009). In June 2010 the family of Claire Allen, who died of cervical cancer at the age of 23 years, presented a petition to Downing Street again calling for the screening age to be lowered (Department of Health 2010).

Screening has received significant attention from health psychology, with the focus primarily upon non-attendance for screening (for example, Neilson and Jones 1998, McCafferey *et al.* 2001) and the investigation of factors that may predict screening attendance/non-attendance including: sociodemographic factors (see Jepson *et al.* 2000); variations in invitation type (Norman and Conner 1992); social cognition models (for example, Bish *et al.* 2000); educational interventions (for example, Wardle *et al.* 1993); and, more recently, variations in information leaflet content (including details about the costs and benefits of screening) to investigate informed choice (Marteau *et al.* 2010). A second area of concern for psychologists, driven by the criterion that screening must not do more harm than good, is the psychological impact of screening on individuals. This has involved investigations into the anxiety associated with receipt of abnormal test results and the requirement to attend for further tests (for example, Brett *et al.* 2005, Orbell *et al.* 2008). Furthermore, the potential impact of receiving negative test results (*i.e.* 'not at risk') has received attention arising from concern that such results could convey a feeling of 'false reassurance' (Pettigrew *et al.* 2000) and in turn trigger a 'certificate of health' effect – meaning that the individual interprets the results as a 'green light' to continue an unhealthy lifestyle (Tymstra and Bieleman 1987).

While there is a crossover between the aspects of screening studied by psychologists and sociologists, for example, studies of the socio-demographic barriers to uptake and the experience and impact of undergoing screening, there are many differences – not least in theoretical and methodological approach, but also in the underlying assumptions and aims. For example, psychologists may use an experimental design to investigate the impact of the manipulation of factors (such as type of information provided) on cognitions, intentions and behaviour related to screening uptake, and thereby provide those overseeing screening programmes with evidence to guide the design of promotional material and invitations to participate in a programme (see, for example, Dillard *et al.* 2011, Marteau *et al.* 2010). In contrast, sociological critiques (such as surveillance and medicalisation) may question a screening programme's materials, and in turn its purpose, as we will describe in the next section.

Sociological work on screening to date

A corpus of sociological work has begun to address population-based medical screening in recent years and has begun to develop important insights that allow us to take a more critical view and move beyond the issue of attendance or non-attendance. This essay is not an exhaustive literature review of sociological work on screening, but rather, provides a broad brush look at some of the more significant sociological insights on screening developed thus far.

One of the central tenets of public health strategies, such as population-based screening, is that non-symptomatic individuals should make their bodies available to health professionals for regular inspection, and that this process needs to be routinised if it is to protect the health of citizens. These assumptions have received much sociological attention, and a sizeable body of sociological work has developed over the last two decades or so that focuses on how health status, and the means for achieving and maintaining good health (including participation in screening programmes), has become a predominant concern of modern society (see, for example, Lupton 1995, Nettleton and Bunton 1995, Petersen and Lupton 1996).

The increased observation and surveillance of the population has been explored at length by David Armstrong (1983, 1993, 1995) and has been termed 'surveillance medicine'. The premise of this concept is that a new model of medicine can be seen as emerging during the 20th century that is concerned with the observation and monitoring of apparently healthy populations. This observation of the seemingly healthy population serves to break down the traditional distinction between those who are healthy and those who are ill. Medicine is no longer concerned simply with the latter; instead, the whole population comes under surveillance and is potentially 'at risk' (Armstrong 1995).

A significant thread of sociological work on screening has drawn on and developed these ideas, often using cervical screening as case material – a particularly amenable example as it involves women being invited at regular intervals through much of their adult life, therefore providing a large and easily accessible pool of potential research participants. Howson

(1998, 1999) has problematised women's attendance for cervical screening and linked this to wider debates about the exercise of power within society. Drawing attention to how much of the previous literature and research on cervical screening had adopted an unproblematic view of attendance (seeing it as a consequence of rational decision making and as morally neutral), Howson argued that the act of attendance for screening needed to be more fully explored and could, in fact, be seen as highly problematic. She argues that it:

> can also be understood as a response to a particular expression of power or set of normative expectations . . . compliance with screening cannot be viewed exclusively as a neutral, if desirable, outcome but as a social practice, which is embedded within a moral framework of responsibility and obligation (1999: 402).

Thus, a key contribution of sociological attention to screening which is transferable beyond this particular case (see, for example, Griffiths *et al.* 2010 on breast cancer screening) has been to draw attention to the ways in which screening attendance can be understood as a response to normative expectations about what constitutes the most sensible and responsible course of action. Attendance at screening may thus be understood as signifying responsible behaviour that demonstrates good citizenship – in Howson's terms, screening attendance becomes a form of 'moral obligation'.

This felt 'moral obligation' to attend for screening has been explored in relation to female embodiment; for example, the obligation that women may feel to respect and look after their bodies (Bush 2000), and the potential to draw on ideas of the surveillance of women's bodies and sexuality in order to understand the cervix as a site of contested control within the female body (McKie 1995). An individual woman's participation within the screening programme may therefore represent more than simply her concern for disease prevention if participation comes to be based more on perceived normalcy and expectation and less on the basis of personal choice. It should be noted, however, that resistance to these powerful discourses is possible (see, for example, N. Armstrong 2007).

There is an increasing focus instigated by the UK National Screening Committee (UK National Screening Committee 2000) on screening, based on informed consent rather than on an expectation of attendance (Jepson *et al.* 2007). The manifest function of information material accompanying invitations to participate in screening is to inform individuals' decision making about participation. However, the tensions between informed choice and ensuring optimal uptake of screening have been discussed within both health policy and medical sociology spheres (Raffle 2001). One immediate issue is what constitutes 'full information' and how this imperative fits with providing information that is accessible to the target audience. Adapting technical information for a generalist lay audience necessarily involves simplification and selectivity. The information provided may also be influenced by a desire to present screening in particular ways. For example, Braun and Gavey (1999) argue that cervical cancer prevention policy in New Zealand largely suppressed sexual risk factor information as policy makers sought to avoid linking cervical cancer and screening to sexual promiscuity or adventurousness in order to avoid potential stigma and maintain attendance levels.

The provision of written information materials (typically in the form of leaflets that accompany invitations) is however likely to be only one part of the much bigger and more complex picture of the factors and issues which influence and inform how people make decisions about whether to have screening, as sociological work across a range of screening types is beginning to show. Pertinent issues include those relating to the technologies or techniques used in screening (see, for example, Chapple *et al.* 2008 on the faecal occult blood test for bowel cancer screening); how individuals think about and understand their own risk of developing a particular condition (see, for example, Pfeffer 2004, N. Armstrong 2005); the possible influence of the wider context in which screening is offered (see, for example, Pilnick 2008, Todorova *et al.* 2006); and how those invited to participate in particularly sensitive or new types of screening act as 'moral pioneers' (Williams *et al.* 2005, Markens *et al.* 2010).

The wider sociological concern with issues of risk and uncertainty has also proved to be fertile ground for those seeking ways into thinking sociologically about screening. For example, Green *et al.* (2002) explored the role that health technologies such as breast cancer screening may play in the 'management' of midlife women's bodies, and the way in which messages about these technologies and their potential are interpreted by women, and Griffiths *et al.* (2006) have used uncertainty as a way of thinking about the issues faced by health professionals in balancing individual and population costs and benefits of screening for breast cancer. In cases where screening has highlighted that there may (potentially) be a problem, the uncertainty experienced by individuals and the ways in which they attempt to understand and cope with this uncertainty has been a particular area of focus; for example, in relation to cervical abnormalities (Blomberg *et al.* 2009, Forss *et al.* 2004, Kavanagh and Broom 1998), prenatal screening (Heyman *et al.* 2006) and newborn screening (Grob 2008).

To summarise: work on the sociology of screening to date has been informed by and contributed to by a range of theories including: surveillance medicine, citizenship and responsibilisation; embodiment; decision making and informed choice; and risk and uncertainty. We now move on to reflect on why this work has not been brought together previously.

What's holding a sociology of screening back?

Despite marked sociological interest in health promotion and preventative interventions more widely during the mid to late 1990s (see, for example, Peterson and Lupton 1996, Nettleton 1995, Burrows *et al.* 1995, Castel 1991, Lupton 1995, D. Armstrong 1993), sociological work on screening can be characterised as fragmented and widely dispersed, making this focused collection of sociological analysis of screening an important step forward in consolidating and stimulating work in this area.

There are a number of possible factors contributing to why a sociology of screening is not further advanced than it currently is. First, at present, the sociological study of screening is largely undertaken within a range of specific sub-disciplines under the broad disciplinary umbrella of sociology. The discipline of sociology of health and illness is the home for much of this work, but work is also going on in other areas of sociology, including science and technology studies; human reproduction; sociology of the body and embodiment; and risk and society. In addition, much sociological work on screening draws on particular ideological or theoretical positions (for example, that may be linked to the sub-discipline in which the work is grounded) or methodological traditions (there is, for example, a body of work on informed choice in relation to screening conducted through conversation analysis). The danger is that this may result in work which speaks primarily to audiences concerned with, or interested in, these theoretical or methodological approaches, rather than having a broader appeal to the wider sociological audience. We would suggest communication across these clusters is not as good as it might be, meaning that this body of work is not yet realising its full potential and has so far failed to become more than the sum of its individual parts.

Secondly, one could argue that the tendency for researchers to focus on specific examples of screening when conducting empirical work leads to their insights largely remaining contained within these case studies. So, for example, while empirical work on different kinds of screening may draw on similar sociological theories and concepts in order to frame and inform the work, the subsequent findings are not always then fed back up to a broader sociological audience where they may contribute to the development and refinement of theoretical and conceptual approaches. Thus, while there are indeed useful pockets of work focusing on a diverse range of screening examples, there is relatively little evidence that these are cross-fertilising or stimulating the production of theoretical approaches that might have purchase across the area of screening as a whole. Many of the theoretical or conceptual ideas that emerge from and within particular examples (such as the management of uncertainty, or feelings of obligation and responsibility) may be applied in other screening contexts and may indeed benefit from the development and refinement this application could bring, but as yet there is little evidence that this is occurring. This may not be a problem unique to a sociology of screening, though, as medical sociology more generally has been characterised as relatively atheoretical (Bird *et al.* 2000, Annandale 1998), and this appeared to be reflected in a comparative analysis of journal content (Seale 2008).

Finally, many sociologically important questions have not yet been addressed either empirically or theoretically by the existing literature, and the agenda for future research is underdeveloped. We turn to this issue in the following section.

Where next for a sociology of screening?

The selection of essays in this collection brings together the work of scholars from different branches of sociology to demonstrate the range of theoretical and methodological approaches currently guiding sociological scrutiny of different aspects of medical screening. We argue that this collection showcases the sociology of screening as it currently stands and that it demonstrates several important recent trends.

First, there is an increasing focus on going beyond individuals' experiences of screening. Some of this (but not all) corresponds with another increase we have noted – in ethnographic approaches (see, for example, the chapters by Kehr, and by Timmermans and Buchbinder). This is in line with the argument that a sociology of screening should not concern itself solely with the experiences of individuals, be they potential or actual patients or health professionals, but that further attention to the infrastructure of screening is required (Singleton 1998). Indeed, as the demand for new technologies increases, sociological scrutiny of these developments, their implementation, and their impacts is vital. The 'bigger picture' questions tackled in essays such as those by Faulkner, by Hogarth, Hopkins and Rodriguez, and by Timmermans and Buchbinder, make important contributions by exploring and critically examining how screening technology is developed and implemented; how knowledge is produced; the roles of key players – both at the 'blunt' end (*i.e.* at the level of policy makers) and the 'sharp' end (for example, in the screening consultation); and the reach of screening programmes. On another level, as globalisation continues to impact on the make-up of a country's population, and health inequalities continue to widen, there will be increasing need to pay attention to the reach of screening programmes and their implications for particular groups within society, for example, as discussed by Kehr.

Secondly, we earlier emphasised the need for studies that do focus on the screening experience to develop and extend theories and concepts that can be more widely applied across the sociology of screening. Gillespie's concept of *measured vulnerability* is a good example, as is Timmermans and Buchbinder's *bridging work* and Hogarth and colleagues' extension of the concept of molecularisation.

In addition to these new directions in the sociological study of screening, it is important to reflect on the continuation and development of established analytical approaches to screening. For example, see the essay by Pilnick and Zayts for a conversation analytic approach to screening consultations and encounters which continues to contribute to our understanding of the key interactional processes involved. Furthermore, pivotal concepts – for example, risk and society, surveillance and embodiment – continue to be drawn upon as demonstrated by the essays in this book. We would argue that as the reach of population-based medical screening grows, so will the range of available foci for a sociology of screening and, in turn, the amount that sociology can contribute.

We turn now to the collection of essays in this book; providing a brief overview of each and highlighting key links between them.

Introduction to the collection

David Armstrong's 'Screening: mapping medicine's temporal spaces' presents a genealogy of population screening. The essay charts the history of the use of the term 'screening' from initial metaphors early in the 20th century, through the first organised programmes identifying disease in the inter-war years, to contemporary debates about the implications and potential harms of screening. Concurrently it maps the associated changing conceptualisation of illness in terms of its temporality and, related to this, the changing nature of the patient from a passive recipient of medical procedures to a subjective and autonomous one.

Armstrong's sources include medical journals, editorials and correspondence; thus, the resulting story follows a trajectory of a phenomenon's beginnings, growth and successful widespread implementation, followed by the emergence of unforeseen implications and dilemmas. It is interesting to contrast this story with the parallel rising demand for screening programmes, evident in the agendas and voices of policy makers, lobbyists and the public.

Armstrong describes the emergence of the 'risk factor' as the focus of screening and the resulting changes in how illness is conceived, in particular in terms of its temporal trajectory. The 'risk factor', and the argument that risk constitutes an illness in and of itself, form the focus of the third chapter, 'The experience of risk as "measured vulnerability": health screening and lay uses of numerical risk' (Gillespie).

Focusing on the cases of high cholesterol and of raised PSA levels, Chris Gillespie uses empirical data to examine how people interpret and experience risk in their everyday lives following receipt of a 'high risk' result. He explores the lay (and sometimes professional) tendency to interpret numerical measures of health, and the importance of numbers not only in the diagnosis of risk but in the management of uncertainty (and vulnerability) arising from that risk. His resulting concept – measured vulnerability – acknowledges the significance that numbers hold in the diagnosis and management of the lived risk experience, as well as the vulnerability to which this use of numerics leads.

A key strength of Gillespie's essay relates to our argument about the need to develop theoretical and conceptual ideas from studying one type of screening that can be applied to a variety of screening contexts. Gillespie goes beyond studying lay experiences of screening from an 'experiences of health and illness' framework, to develop a concept that is applicable to medical screening in general, which thus becomes a key concept in the sociology of medical screening to be refined by future work. This strength is also demonstrated by the next chapter from Stefan Timmermans and Mara Buchbinder, 'Expanded newborn screening: articulating the ontology of diseases with bridging work in the clinic'. While Gillespie's essay focuses on the uncertainty experienced by lay people following receipt of numerical screening test results, Timmermans and Buchbinder explore another type of uncertainty that can arise from the implementation of a screening programme – uncertainty in knowledge about the condition being screened for, as experienced by clinicians and parents of children identified with a metabolic disease following newborn screening.

Timmermans and Buchbinder unpack one of Wilson and Jungner's (1968) criteria for screening – that the natural history of the condition, including development from latent to declared disease, should be adequately understood – by demonstrating how a screening programme itself can transform knowledge about a disease. In their ethnographic study of a clinical centre for metabolic-genetic disorders, they demonstrate how the implementation of population-based newborn screening for medium chain acyl-CoA dehydrogenase deficiency (MCADD) led to changes in knowledge about the condition, its variants and anomalies. They introduce the concept of 'bridging work' to describe how clinicians reconcile this gap in knowledge; this comprised the team collectively engaging in continuous learning about the disease and developing procedures to manage the changed ontology, while practically – in the clinic – adapting patient care in light of the changed knowledge.

Next, we take a step back and consider aspects related to what can be conceptualised as the 'blunt' end of screening – the development, initiation, implementation and evaluation of screening programmes. The goal of finding testing technology with optimal sensitivity and specificity is a key aspect of this; and a focus on the companies that develop these, and the scientific assessment and governance of these, unsurprisingly attracts sociological attention. Conditions for which no systematic population-screening programme is currently in place, but that have received considerable scrutiny from policymakers provide a particularly useful case study. A pertinent example, which has been the subject of controversy in the UK, is the screening and detection of localised prostate cancer, and this is the focus of Alex Faulkner's chapter 'Resisting the screening imperative: patienthood, populations and politics in prostate cancer detection technologies for the UK'. Faulkner outlines the controversy and uncertainty surrounding the issue and describes recent technological developments including PSA testing, the search for genetic biomarkers and genome-wide association tests. He analyses the response to these developments by drawing on theories of risk and governance, the sociology of technology governance and the sociology of technology expectations. In doing so he charts the different modes of resistance demonstrated by public health policymakers and reflects on the shift in policy to an 'informed choice' framework.

The search for genetic and genomic detection technology, and its relationship with established testing technology, is not limited to prostate cancer. Stuart Hogarth, Michael Hopkins and Victor Rodriguez track the development of gene-based diagnostic testing for cervical cancer detection in their chapter, 'A molecular monopoly? HPV testing, the Pap smear and the molecularisation of cervical screening in the USA'. While Faulkner reflects on key players in terms of the policy, regulation and governance of testing technologies, Hogarth and colleagues narrow their focus onto a diagnostics company, Digene, and critically examine the company's development and marketing of a molecular alternative to the Pap smear. Using a science and technology studies framework, Hogarth and colleagues extend the concept of molecularisation to examine and illustrate how the process of genomic molecularisation plays out in this context of screening. They use their findings to demonstrate a cumulative process with the new technology integrating with the established method. Secondly, when examining corporatisation, they demonstrate the growing importance of diagnostics companies in developing and disseminating innovation in this area.

The next chapter continues the focus on key players in the implementation of screening programmes. As described by Armstrong, the drive to diagnose, prevent and eradicate tuberculosis (TB) triggered the first instances of screening. While population-wide screening for TB is no longer required in developed countries, targeted TB screening in migrant populations is the focus of Janina Kehr's chapter, 'Blind spots and adverse conditions of care: screening migrants for tuberculosis in France and Germany'. In her multi-site ethnographic study of TB prevention centres, Kehr critically examines each country's guidelines to explore how they are enacted on the ground in each case. In doing so, she highlights problems and implications throughout the process – from the collection of epidemiological data (particularly in terms of what is not collected), through to the treatment of cases identified through screening (and the difficulty of ensuring treatment completion). In distinguishing her findings from previous studies of TB screening and of public health practice, she argues that, rather than being stigmatising and surveying, these two examples of targeted migrant TB screening are exclusionary through being ineffective and constrained by political measures. She argues that TB screening is political in nature, and concerned with controlling disease not treating the people who have it.

The next few essays explore different aspects of what we conceptualise as the 'sharp end' of screening – sociological studies of the screening consultation. The first two chapters focus on prenatal screening consultations. First, Alison Pilnick and Olga Zayts examine the interactional processes involved in decision making following a 'high risk' screening test result for fetal abnormality in their essay, '"Let's have it tested first": choice and circumstances in decision-making following positive antenatal screening in Hong Kong'. Reflecting on debates about the principle of non-directiveness in antenatal screening, they point out that the interactional nature of antenatal screening means that directiveness is likely to be an unintended outcome. Indeed, through conversation analysis (CA) of videoed consultations, they argue that the visibility of a woman's socioeconomic background or circumstances can impact on how a consultation is played out, including how decisions are made, and how they are accepted or challenged by the counselling professionals.

In the essay 'Representing and intervening: "doing" good care in first trimester knowledge production and decision-making', Nete Schwennesen and Lene Koch demonstrate not only that non-directiveness is not achieved in prenatal counselling, but also argue that complete non-directiveness in these consultations would not constitute good care. In their ethnographic study in Danish ultrasound clinics, they explore processes of knowledge production and decision making at two key passage points of first trimester prenatal risk assessment (FTPRA) – the performance of the ultrasound scan, and the communication of the risk figure and subsequent discussion about the woman's decision. They argue that sonographers employ three different modes of 'doing good care' instead of non-directiveness to achieve the same aim of providing an ethical and accountable approach to prenatal counselling: attuning knowledge and expectations throughout; allowing space for resistance; and providing situated influence in the context of uncertainty.

As we have seen, uncertainty is an implicit theme running through all of the empirical essays in this collection. Schwennesen and Koch demonstrate how women use the FTPRA consultation to deal with this uncertainty – by gaining knowledge about the likely risk to their fetus and the meaning of the risk figure – but often also to ask for guidance in making a decision following receipt of such complex risk knowledge. In the final chapter in this book, Julie Roberts demonstrates a different use of screening; in her chapter on privately-provided four-dimensional bonding scans during pregnancy, she explores a new social practice of using screening technologies for non-medical purposes.

Ultrasound is routinely used within antenatal care and, in the UK, the NHS Fetal Anomaly Screening Programme includes an ultrasound scan at about 18–20 weeks which may detect structural abnormalities such as spina bifida. As Roberts outlines, however, the boundaries between the medical and social components of this are blurred as parents-to-be are frequently at least as, if not more, interested in 'seeing' and 'getting to know' the baby as they are with the clinical significance of the scan. Drawing on ethnographic research in the UK, ' "Wakey wakey baby": narrating four-dimensional (4D) bonding scans' explores the issues and tensions raised when this screening technology moves outside the clinical setting and begins to be used for social rather than medical purposes.

Conclusion

As we have said, our aims for this book are threefold: to reflect on the sociology of screening to date; to suggest ways in which the sociology of screening could move forward; and to bring together a collection of new essays demonstrating current sociological work on screening. We have addressed the first two aims in this introductory chapter. The rest of this book addresses our third aim and showcases a range of work that constitutes the sociology of screening as it currently stands. The varied contributions address a range of issues using several different theoretical and methodological approaches. Taken together, they both demonstrate current sociological concerns around screening and make clear recommendations for future sociological work in this area.

Contemporary debates about population-based medical screening are currently taking place across a variety of forums, and involve diverse stakeholders, from patients' groups to policy makers and health service managers, and from laboratory scientists to clinicians (as demonstrated by Faulkner). Many of these debates are very heated, with frequent claims and counter-claims made to support particular positions and interests. It almost goes without saying that the kinds of evidence that particular groups draw upon and cite in support of their positions and demands can vary enormously, with a common juxtaposition being discernible between personal experience or understanding of a disease on the one hand and epidemiological study and technical principles on the other (see, for example, Barker and Galardi 2011, N. Armstrong and Murphy 2008, N. Armstrong *et al.* 2010, Wieser 2010, Lehoux *et al.* 2010). Developing a rigorous and focused sociology of screening will help to invigorate and inform these debates, in particular by affording deeper recognition of the social and ethical implications of screening, and will contribute to the evidence base on which policy and practice are founded.

Acknowledgements

We are grateful to Elizabeth Murphy, Mary Dixon-Woods, Julia Lawton and Hannah Bradby for helpful comments and suggestions on an earlier draft of this essay. We would also like to thank the authors of the nine chapters we have brought together for this book.

Note

1   Full details of the UK National Screening Committee criteria for screening programmes can be found at: http://www.screening.nhs.uk/criteria

References

Advisory Committee on Cervical Screening (2009) Minutes of extraordinary meeting to re-examine current policy on cervical screening for women aged 20–24 years taking account of any new evidence and to make recommendations to the National Cancer Director and Ministers. Available at: http://www.cancerscreening.nhs.uk/cervical/cervical-review-minutes-20090519.pdf

Annandale, E. (1998) *The Sociology of Health and Medicine: a Critical Introduction*. Cambridge: Polity Press.

Armstrong, D. (1983) *Political Anatomy of the Body*. Cambridge: Cambridge University Press.

Armstrong, D. (1993) Public health spaces and the fabrication of identity, *Sociology*, 27, 3, 393–410.

Armstrong, D. (1995) The rise of surveillance medicine, *Sociology of Health and Illness*, 17, 393–404.

Armstrong, N. (2005) Resistance through risk: women and cervical cancer screening, *Health, Risk and Society*, 7, 161–76.

Armstrong, N. (2007) Discourse and the individual in cervical cancer screening, *Health: An Interdisciplinary Journal for the Social Study of Health, Illness and Medicine*, 11, 69–85.

Armstrong, N. and Murphy, E. (2008) Weaving meaning? An exploration of the interplay between lay and professional understandings of cervical cancer risk, *Social Science and Medicine*, 67, 1074–82.

Armstrong, N. Dixon-Woods, M. and Murphy, E. (2010) Age criteria for cervical screening in England: qualitative study of women's views, Department of Health Sciences, University of Leicester Working Papers Series No.10:01 Available at: http://hdl.handle.net/2381/8782

Barker, K.K. and Galardi, T.R. (2011) Dead by 50: lay expertise and breast cancer screening, *Social Science and Medicine*, 72, 1351–58.

Baum, M., McCartney, M., Thornton, H. and Bewley, S. (2009) Breast cancer screening peril: negative consequences of the breast screening programme, *The Times*, 19 Feb.

Bird, C.E., Conrad, P. and Fremont, A.M. (2000) Medical sociology at the millennium. In Bird, C.E., Conrad, P. and Fremont, A.M. (eds) *Handbook of Medical Sociology*: 5th Edition. New Jersey: Prentice Hall.

Bish, A., Sutton, S. and Golombok, S. (2000) Predicting uptake of a routine cervical smear test: a comparison of the health belief model and the theory of planned behaviour, *Psychology and Health*, 15, 35–50.

Braun, V. and Gavey, N. (1999) 'With the best of reasons': cervical cancer prevention policy and the suppression of risk factor information, *Social Science and Medicine*, 48, 1463–74.

Brett, J., Bankhead, C., Henderson, B., Watson, E. and Austoker, J. (2005) The psychological impact of mammographic screening: a systematic review, *Psycho-oncology*, 14, 917–38.

Bush, J. (2000) 'It's just part of being a woman': cervical screening, the body and femininity, *Social Science and Medicine*, 50, 3, 429–44.

Burrows, R., Nettleton, S. and Bunton, R. (1995) Sociology and health promotion: health, risk and consumption under late modernism. In Bunton, R., Nettleton, S. and Burrows, R. (eds) *The Sociology of Health Promotion: Critical Analyses of Consumption, Lifestyle and Risk*. London: Routledge.

Castel, R. (1991) From dangerousness to risk. In Burchell, G., Gordon, C. and Miller, P. (eds) *The Foucault Effect*. London: Harvester Wheatsheaf.

Chapple, A., Ziebland, S., Hewitson P. and McPherson, A. (2008) What affects the uptake of screening for bowel cancer using a faecal occult blood test (FOBt): a qualitative study, *Social Science and Medicine*, 66, 2425–35.

Cole, A. (2010) UK patients are given advice on private screening, *BMJ*, 341, c5394.

Cox, S.M. and McKellin, W. (1999) 'There's this thing in our family': predictive testing and the construction of risk for Huntington Disease, *Sociology of Health and Illness*, 21, 622–46.

Davison, C., Macintyre, S. and Davey Smith, G. (1994) The potential social impact of predictive genetic testing for susceptibility to common chronic diseases: a review and proposed research agenda, *Sociology of Health and Illness*, 16, 340–71.

Department of Health (2009) *Free NHS Health Check: Helping you Prevent heart Disease, Stroke, Diabetes and Kidney Disease*. London: Department of Health.

Department of Health (2010) Comment on calls to lower cervical cancer screening age. Available at: http://www.dh.gov.uk/en/MediaCentre/Statements/DH_116591 (accessed 31.8.2011)

Dillard, A.J., Ferrer, R.A., Ubel, P.A. and Fagerlin, A. (2011) Risk perception measures' associations with behavior intentions, affect, and cognition following colon cancer screening messages, *Health Psychology*, 1 August 2011, no pagination specified, doi: 10.1037/a0024787 ⟨http://psycnet.apa.org/doi/10.1037/a0024787⟩.

Gøtzsche, P.C. and Nielsen, M. (2009) Screening for breast cancer with mammography, *Cochrane Database of Systematic Reviews*, 1, CD001877.

Green, E., Thompson, E. and Griffiths, F. (2002) Narratives of risk: women at midlife, medical 'experts' and health technologies, *Health, Risk and Society*, 4, 273–86.

Griffiths, F., Green, E. and Bendelow, G. (2006) Health professionals, their medical interventions and uncertainty: A study focusing on women at midlife, *Social Science and Medicine*, 62, 1078–90.

Griffiths, F., Bendelow, G., Green, E. and Palmer, J. (2010) Screening for breast cancer: Medicalization, visualization and the embodied experience, *Health*, 14, 653–68.

Grob, R. (2008) Is my sick child healthy? Is my healthy child sick?: changes in parental experiences of cystic fibrosis in the age of expanded newborn screening, *Social Science and Medicine*, 67, 1056–64.

Hallowell, N. (1999) Doing the right thing: genetic risk and responsibility, *Sociology of Health and Illness*, 21, 5, 597–621.

Hallowell, N., Arden-Jones, A., Eeles, R., Foster, C., Lucassen, A., Moynihan, C. and Watson, M. (2006) Guilt, blame and responsibility: men's understanding of their role in the transmission of BRCA1/2 mutations within their family, *Sociology of Health and Illness*, 28, 969–88.

Heyman, B., Lewando Hundt, G., Sandall, J., Spencer, K., Williams, C., Grellier, R. and Pitson, L. (2006) On being at higher risk: prenatal screening for chromosomal anomalies, *Social Science and Medicine*, 62, 2360–72.

Howson, A. (1998) Embodied obligation: the female body and health surveillance. In Nettleton, S. and Watson, J. (eds) *The Body in Everyday Life*. London: Routledge

Howson, A. (1999) Cervical screening, compliance and moral obligation, *Sociology of Health and Illness*, 21, 4, 401–25.

Howson, A. (2001) Locating uncertainties in cervical screening, *Health, Risk and Society*, 3, 167–79.

Jepson, R., Clegg, A., Forbes, C., Lewis, R., Sowden, A. and Kleijnen, J. (2000) The determinants of screening uptake and interventions for increasing uptake: a systematic review, *Health Technology Assessment*, 4, 14.

Jepson, R.G., Hewison, J., Thompson, A. and Weller, D. (2007) Patient perspectives on information and choice in cancer screening: A qualitative study in the UK, *Social Science and Medicine*, 65, 890–99.

Jutel, A. and Nettleton, S. (2011) Towards a sociology of diagnosis: reflections and opportunities, *Social Science and Medicine*, 73, 6, 793–800.

Kavanagh, A.M. and Broom, D.H. (1998) Embodied risk: my body, myself? *Social Science and Medicine*, 46, 437–44.

Lehoux, P., Denis, J.-L., Rock, M., Hivon, M. and Tailliez, M. (2010) How medical specialists appraise three controversial health innovations: scientific, clinical and social arguments, *Sociology of Health and Illness*, 32, 123–39.

Lupton, D. (1995) *The Imperative of Health*. London: Sage.

Markens, S., Browner, C.H. and Preloran, H.M. (2010) Interrogating the dynamics between power, knowledge and pregnant bodies in amniocentesis decision making, *Sociology of Health and Illness*, 32, 37–56.

Marteau, T.M., Mann, E., Prevost, A.T., Vasconcelos, J.C., Kellar, I., Sanderson, S., Parker, M., Griffin, S., Sutton, S. and Kinmonth, A.-L. (2010) Impact of an informed choice invitation on uptake of screening for diabetes in primary care (DICISION): randomised trial, *BMJ*, 340, 1176.

Mayor, S. (2010) Critics attack new NHS breast screening leaflet for failing to address harms, *BMJ*, 341: c7267.

McCaffery, K., Borril, J., Williamson, S., Taylor, T., Sutton, S., Atkin, W. and Wardle J. (2001) Declining the offer of flexible sigmoidoscopy screening for bowel cancer: a qualitative investigation of the decision-making process, *Social Science and Medicine*, 53, 679–91.

McKie, L. (1995) The art of surveillance or reasonable prevention? The case of cervical screening, *Sociology of Health and Illness*, 17, 4, 441–57.

McPherson, K. (2010) Should we screen for breast cancer? *BMJ*, 340, c310.

National Screening Committee. (2011) UK screening portal. Available from: http://www.screening.nhs.uk

Neilson, A. and Jones, R. (1998) Women's lay knowledge of cervical cancer/cervical screening: accounting for non-attendance at cervical screening clinics, *Journal of Advanced Nursing*, 28, 571–75.

Nettleton, S. (1995) *The Sociology of Health and Illness*. Cambridge: Polity Press.

Nettleton, S. and Bunton, R. (1995) Sociological critiques of health promotion. In Bunton, R., Burrows, R. and Nettleton, S. (eds) *The Sociology of Health Promotion*. London: Routledge.

NHS Cancer Screening Programmes (2011a) http://www.cancerscreening.nhs.uk/breastscreen/cost.html (accessed 31.8.2011).

NHS Cancer Screening Programmes (2011b) http://www.cancerscreening.nhs.uk/cervical/about-cervical-screening.html#cost (accessed 31.8.2011).

Norman, P. and Conner, M. (1992) Health checks in General Practice, *Family Practice*, 9, 481–87.

Orbell, S., O'Sullivan, I., Parker, R., Steele, B., Campbell, C. and Weller, D. (2008) Illness representations and coping following an abnormal colorectal cancer screening result, *Social Science and Medicine*, 67, 1465–74.

Petersen, A. and Lupton, D. (1996) *The New Public Health*. London: Sage.

Pettigrew, M., Sowden, A., Lister-Sharp, D. and Wright, K. (2000) False-negative results in screening programmes: systematic review of impact and implications, *Health Technology Assessment*, 4, 5, 1–33.

Pfeffer, N. (2004) Screening for breast cancer: candidacy and compliance, *Social Science and Medicine*, 58, 151–60.

Pilnick, A. (2008) 'It's something for you both to think about': choice and decision making in nuchal translucency screening for Down's syndrome, *Sociology of Health and Illness*, 30, 4, 511–30.

Polzer, J., Mercer, S.L. and Goel, V. (2002) Blood is thicker than water: genetic testing as citizenship through familial obligation and the management of risk, *Critical Public Health*, 12, 2, 153–68.

Raffle, A.E. (2001) Information about screening – is it to achieve high uptake or to ensure informed choice? *Health Expectations*, 4, 92–8.

Raspberry, K. and Skinner, D. (2011) Enacting genetic responsibility: experiences of mothers who carry the fragile X gene, *Sociology of Health and Illness*, 33, 420–33.

Reed, K. (2009) 'It's them faulty genes again': women, men and the gendered nature of genetic responsibility in prenatal blood screening, *Sociology of Health and Illness*, 31, 343–59.

Seale, C. (2008) Mapping the field of medical sociology: a comparative analysis of journals, *Sociology of Health and Illness*, 30, 677–95.

Singleton, V. (1998) Stabilizing instabilities: the role of the laboratory in the United Kingdom cervical screening programme. In Berg, M. and Mol, A. (eds) *Differences in Medicine: Unravelling Practices, Techniques and Bodies*. Durham: Duke University Press.

Steinberg, D.L. (1996) Languages of risk: genetic encryptions of the female body: Women, a Cultural Review, Volume 7.

Todorova, I.L.G., Baban, A., Balabanova, D., Panayotova, Y. and Bradley, J. (2006) Providers' constructions of the role of women in cervical cancer screening in Bulgaria and Romania, *Social Science and Medicine*, 63, 776–87.

Tymstra, T. and Bieleman, B. (1987) The psychosocial impact of mass screening for cardiovascular risk factors, *Family Practice*, 4, 4, 287–90.

UK National Screening Committee. (2000) Second Report of the UK National Screening Committee. Available from: http://www.dh.gov.uk/prod_consum_dh/groups/dh_digitalassets/@dh/@en/documents/digitalasset/dh_4014560.pdf

Wardle, J., Williamson, S., McCaffery, K., Sutton, S., Taylor, T., Edwards, R. and Atkin, W. (2003) Increasing attendance at colorectal cancer screening: testing the efficacy of a mailed, psychoeducational intervention in a community sample of older adults, *Health Psychology*, 22, 99–105.

Watson, M.S., Lloyd-Puryear, M.A., Mann, M.Y., Ronaldo, P. and Howell, R.R. (2006) Newborn Screening: Toward a Uniform Screening Panel and System, *Genetics in Medicine*, 8, 5 (Supplement), 12S.

Wieser, B. (2010) Public accountability of newborn screening: Collective knowing and deciding, *Social Science and Medicine*, 70, 926–33.

Williams, C., Sandall, J., Lewando-Hundt, G., Heyman, B., Spencer, K. and Grellier, R. (2005) Women as moral pioneers? Experiences of first trimester antenatal screening, *Social Science and Medicine*, 61, 1983–92.

Wilson, J.M.G. and Jungner, G. (1968) Principles and practice of screening for disease. Public health paper No. 34. Geneva: World Health Organisation. Available from: http://www.who.int/bulletin/volumes/86/4/07-050112BP.pdf

Yamey, G. and Wilkes, M. (2002) The PSA storm: Questioning cancer screening can be a risky business in America, *British Medical Journal*, 324, 431.

2

Screening: mapping medicine's temporal spaces
David Armstrong

A century or so ago 'screening the patient' would probably have referred to the use of curtains around the patient's hospital bed to provide privacy for a medical procedure. In the 1950s, it marked the brave new world of testing the population for the early stages of disease. Nowadays, it is likely to be a site of contestation over whether it confers benefits or harms. This chapter attempts to map these changing uses of the term and the debates which have surrounded its deployment, from its first appearance in the inter-war years of the 20th century, through its period of ascendancy in the post-war years, to its more turbulent history in the early 21st century. In doing so the chapter identifies underlying changes in the temporal dimension of illness, of which screening is simply one manifestation.

The role of population screening within healthcare has been of interest to doctors, patients, lay groups, lobbyists, and other healthcare professionals, among others, but the analysis in this chapter is based primarily on debates within medicine – the relationship with these other discourses is briefly discussed in the final section. Medical engagement with screening was accessed by examining contemporary medical journal articles, editorials and correspondence. Major medical journals are now digitalised and word searchable from their first issues, so they were used to identify when, and in what context, the notion of medical screening was separated from earlier different uses of the term. The subsequent expansion of the use of screening as a routine medical procedure was tracked through a range of medical journals published in both the UK and US supplemented by PubMed searches. Trends were charted in Excel and these were corroborated using Google Ngrams which word searches over five million books (Michel and Shen *et al.* 2011). These trends were then explored in more detail, in particular looking for evidence of changes in the meaning or context of use of screening and related constructs. This process also facilitated the choice of illustrative material used to underpin the chapter's narrative.

The screen

Discovery of the diagnostic value of X-rays at the very end of the 19th century was followed by their application in routine clinical practice. The fact that the radiographic image was viewed on a screen meant that the terms 'screen' and 'screening' began to be applied to

The Sociology of Medical Screening, First Edition. Edited by Natalie Armstrong and Helen Eborall.
Chapters © 2012 The Authors. Book Compilation © 2012 Foundation for the Sociology of Health
& Illness / Blackwell Publishing Ltd. Published 2012 by Blackwell Publishing Ltd.

patients undergoing X-ray examination. In a study of the value of X-rays in the diagnosis of lung cancer, for example, it was observed that 'The movement of the ribs during inspiration may be plainly seen by means of the screen . . . [though in this case] the physical signs were so conclusive that screening does not afford the physician any real assistance' (Lawson and Crombie 1903: 212).

One of the main reasons for X-raying a patient was to identify the then relatively common disease of tuberculosis. Tuberculosis usually presented clinically with weight loss and haemoptysis (coughing of blood) only after the disease had been well established; X-ray examination, however, could detect the very early stages of the disease before its presence became overt. The threat of 'latent tuberculosis' was a particular hazard for people living close together, such as school-children, for whom cross-infection was a real risk and 'screening of the chest and the inspection of films' gave useful diagnostic information (Conference Report 1931: 28). During the inter-war years attempts to identify latent tuberculosis, such as the Massachusetts Children's Tuberculosis Program, involved radiological screening of all those children found to have a higher risk of having the disease, as indicated by a positive response to tuberculin challenge (Wakefield 1930), but later studies began to use X-rays as the first diagnostic sieve. A study of the prevalence of tuberculosis in medical students, for example, carried out at the University of Pennsylvania in 1931 (Hetherington *et al.* 1931), involved X-ray screening all students.

The search for latent tuberculosis was characterised by two related features. The first was the idea of early diagnosis. Treatment options for tuberculosis were few, but it was still a communicable disease, and identification of latent disease was of some importance for the further spread of the disease. The consequent challenge was to recognise the disease as early as possible in its natural history and X-ray 'screening' provided an enabling technology. Secondly, the identification of latent cases implied examining otherwise normal populations which exhibited no symptoms of tubercle infection. These two key elements of screening, which informed its growth and spread in the second half of the 20th century, can therefore be discerned in the early attempts to track tuberculosis in the population. It was also only a small step for the word 'screening', initially derived from a characteristic of the X-ray process, to become shorthand for the process of medically examining 'normal' populations for latent disease; but that step was reinforced by parallel developments in the field of public health.

The second derivation of the terms screen/screening which informs modern usage came from public health. In the late 19th century various medical discoveries alerted doctors to the dangers of vector-borne diseases, particularly those carried by flies and mosquitoes. One way of protecting against the mosquito was to use screens or meshes over windows and doors – hence the frequent exploration of the best way of 'screening a building' in the early decades of the 20th century. Public health also borrowed another meaning of screening from manufacturing and extractive industries where it referred to the use of some sort of sieve to separate larger particles from smaller ones. In sanitary work, for example, it was not uncommon to 'screen' various forms of effluent: 'coarse screening' was one way of protecting rivers from gross pollution (Lancet Editorial 1899), or, as Soper (1914) noted, some of the most objectionable substances in effluent 'which look offensive in the water' (1914: 1091) could easily be removed by use of screens.

In the inter-war years the idea of a metaphorical mesh or screen began to be used to describe the process of separating out abnormality from normality amongst school-children. The application of screening to children reflected the same imperative that drove the early detection of tuberculosis: as the child was growing, any unidentified disease or abnormality might cause future harms unless it was detected early and 'corrected'. In the US in the 1920s, for example, Buck (1925) described the role of a preliminary 'screening' inspection (she used the word in quotation marks given the novel application of the term) of children by the teacher prior to the school medical examination. In the same year Champion (1925) also described the preliminary sifting of school-children prior to a detailed medical inspection, and questioned whether it should be designated as a screening or diagnostic process, while at the same time pointing out that the word screening in this context was not in general use.

Routine screening of children for sight and hearing emerged as applications for the new approach to diagnosis, which targeted normal populations rather than patients presenting with symptoms (Oak 1942), but one of the earliest specific diseases to be 'screened out' was tuberculosis (Dugan 1932, AJPH Editorial 1932). There was a clear parallel with the 'screening' undertaken using radiography in the hospital earlier in the century, in that both uses of the term referred to identifying the same disease. When 'mass radiography' was later offered to adult populations as a means of screening for tuberculosis (Bentley and Leitner 1940), the X-ray and the sieve derivations of 'screening' finally coalesced.

Controlling future threats

The Second World War provided ideal conditions for the spread of screening technology. It had been usual for new recruits to undergo a medical examination to assess overall fitness for active service and during wartime this examination was increasingly supplemented with formal screening programmes. Those diseases for which there were screening tests, such as tuberculosis and syphilis, provided exemplars of how the technology could be deployed: a defined population, preferably captive to the extent that their compliance was assured, and a test which could identify latent disease. Mass radiography had already been evaluated in civilian populations in many countries in the inter-war years (Bentley and Leitner 1940) but in wartime it took on a new urgency. Cooper (1940), for example, described how 22,000 men underwent X-ray examination/screening in the Australian army in early 1940. Later reports claimed that screening had reduced the spread and overall incidence of tuberculosis in the armed forces (Long and Lew 1945).

The other communicable diseases with high salience since the early 20th century were syphilis and gonorrhoea but these achieved an even higher profile in wartime. Lang (1941) observed that the sickness in the US Navy caused by venereal disease was equivalent to the complement of 11 battleships infected at some time during that year. New screening programmes were therefore established to identify 'latent' disease (Robinson 1941) and new tests were analysed which might be used as a 'screening agency' for blood samples in the identification of syphilis (Webb and Sellers 1943).

The third important screening programme introduced in the armed forces was for psychiatric illness. Memories of shell-shock from WWI led to concerns for the mental state of new recruits, given the risks to other soldiers on the battlefield by those unable to cope with warfare. Unlike the programmes for screening tuberculosis and syphilis, there was little pre-war civilian experience in psychiatric screening so new tests had to be devised to detect recruits at risk. As these tests had the purpose of triaging recruits to identify those needing a more formal psychiatric assessment, they needed to be simple and easy to administer. Psychiatric status could not be measured by biological titration, so a new technology, the screening questionnaire, was developed and refined to supplement – and in part replace – the psychiatrist's assessment. Indeed, such was the perceived power of screening mental state that it became an important tool in assessing all military personnel (Perrot 1944, 1945).

Diagnosis in routine clinical practice had identified pathologies which, in the main, were a burden for the individual; yet there were a number of diseases which because of their communicable nature also posed a threat to others. Early diagnosis of these latter diseases, and their treatment if possible, could therefore be of community as well as individual benefit, and it was this insight which underpinned early attempts to promote screening. Wartime conditions heightened awareness of these threats beyond the individual and hastened the deployment of screening programmes in the armed forces. Since the early 20th century, tuberculosis had been characterised as a disease of interpersonal contact (as against poor sanitary conditions in the 19th century) and the major threat was from 'carriers' in the population who unknowingly could infect others; the dangers to soldiers working closely together were clear. Equally, a single case of syphilis could spread rapidly on some far-off posting if its potential danger was not identified and managed by initial screening. Psychiatric disease, though non-communicable, could also pose a potential danger to others on active service when working together was so important.

The screening of new recruits was extended to encompass tests developed for the school medical examination (for vision and hearing, for example). These tests still carried echoes of danger-to-others which characterised the main screening programmes, as it was the child who threatened the future adult; in fact many of the reasons for rejecting recruits as unfit for active service were childhood diseases and 'abnormalities'. In a novel analysis linking the results of childhood and wartime screening, Ciocco (1945) showed that the growth trajectories mapped in the child were predictive of subsequent military fitness identified in the soldier. The temporal relationship between the child and the young man was further illustrated by problems such as poor dental health, rheumatic fever, eye defects and orthopaedic impairments (like flat feet) which caused recruits to be rejected. These findings reinforced the need for better childhood screening so as to enable earlier identification of abnormalities and avoidance of later problems (Robinson 1941, Shepard et al. 1944).

By the 1940s the inverted commas which often accompanied the use of the term 'screening' to denote its metaphorical use appeared less frequently. Occasionally authors felt compelled to say what it meant ('In screening the attempt is not merely to sift out and discard . . . The word "screening" designates an attempt to obtain an individual picture of each person, whether his place is to be in the Armed Forces or in the industrial army' (Dunbar 1945: 121)), but it was rapidly becoming the accepted descriptor for triaging latent and early manifestations of disease in large numbers of apparently healthy people (Rowntree 1944).

Post-war extension of screening

After the Second World War, mass radiography for tuberculosis was extended to the whole population (Wilson 1946) and surveillance of the growing child was further reinforced (Capon 1950). In addition, the idea that serious disease of later adult life might lie latent in earlier years was extended to the civilian population. Studies of rising death rates from cardiovascular disease revealed widespread lesions in the coronary arteries of young soldiers killed in the Korean War (Enos et al. 1953) leading to calls for screening for latent heart disease in young civilian populations (James 1955). And as the temporal dimension of illness expanded across the lifespan, diseases of older adults began to appear suitable targets for screening. Cases of unsuspected diabetes, for example, were reported as extremely common and whole communities – state and local health departments as well as voluntary and private agencies – could be mobilised as part of the screening effort (JAMA Editorial 1950,

Wilkerson and Ford 1949, Wilkerson *et al.* 1955). Equally, cancer detection clinics, which had first begun to emerge in the US in the 1930s, received post-war impetus from the American Cancer Society, the US Public Health Service and many local health departments (Jones and Cameron 1947, Deibert 1948). Development of cervical smears (which later evolved into the 'pap test' for cervical cancer) (Papanicolaou and Traut 1943) encouraged exploration of cell smear methods for diagnosing other cancers at an early stage (Papanicolaou 1948).

With these new techniques and new targets the decades following WWII were marked by the enthusiastic promotion of screening. Who could argue with its logic or its aim? 'Screening for a disease has a most attractive goal – to find the patient in the early stages of a chronic process and to interrupt its dismal natural course' (Carroll 1976: 646). This was a revolutionary method for replacing the usual symptomatic patient with the 'supposedly well person' (Freemont-Smith 1953) as the focus of healthcare. Chapman (1949) suggested that a screening examination of 1,000 apparently well persons over the age of 15 for syphilis, diabetes, glaucoma, anaemia, tuberculosis, obesity, visual defects, hearing loss, hypertension and heart disease would result in the finding of 976 instances of these diseases. As 12 years' experience at the Tulane University Cancer Detection Clinic confirmed, the value of screening was clear when out of over 10,000 'apparently healthy subjects' 92% were shown to have either organic or functional disease (malignancy being detected in 77 patients) (Schenthal 1960).

Screening was concerned with detecting disease as early as possible in its natural history, the better to be able to alter its subsequent course. The earliest opportunities for detection lay in screening the asymptomatic patient, before the well person experienced illness and chose to present to the doctor (Sisson 1957, Hubbard 1957). Consequently, screening reached out into the community whether through taking the 'clinic' to the home, the street or the factory or by inviting normal populations to visit healthcare settings. The main constraint on screening was the apparently limited number of diseases which had a sufficiently long timeline to enable early manifestations to be identified. An acute disease, for instance, or one with short prodromal features, offered little opportunity for detection through population screening. The potential remit of screening was therefore considerably extended when chronic illness emerged as a major clinical problem. The pre-war identification of chronic illness and the post-war rapid expansion in its perceived importance mapped on perfectly to the surveillance agenda (see Figure 1). In the post-war years, screening and chronic illness became two sides of the same coin in that diseases which could be

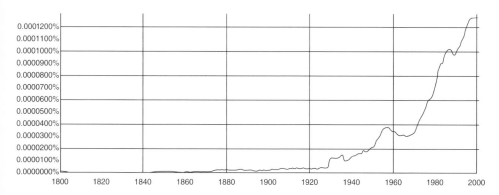

Figure 1 *'Chronic illness' in Google Ngrams. The graph shows the frequency of keywords in a given year as a proportion of the total number of words in the database for that year (Michel et al. 2011)*

characterised as having a temporal trajectory could, in their turn, be captured by the new screening technologies (Halverson *et al.* 1949, JAMA Editorial 1950, Levin 1951, Holmes and Bowden 1951).

The increasing temporalisation of illness in the post-war years, especially through the recognition of the importance of chronic illness, reinforced the significance of prevention: if disease had a developmental timeline then, in principle, it may be possible to delay or halt its progression. The term 'primary prevention' had been used by Dale in 1932 ('Several of the great life-destroying plagues had been banished by a primary prevention' 1932: 1152) but it was only in the 1950s that preventive activity became routinely divided into 'primary prevention' and 'secondary prevention', the latter, which embraced screening, being concerned with stopping early disease progressing further. A decade later, the term 'tertiary prevention' was introduced to describe the rest of clinical activity which could be construed as managing established disease to prevent it getting worse. Post-war medicine therefore mapped out a prevention landscape, a vision of numerous disease timelines which could be targeted at any point so that subsequent illness could be forestalled. Screening was a key component of this wider strategy as it promised to identify and manage disease early in its temporal trajectory; yet this population project was to be undermined by the fragmentation of the temporal space in which illness was located.

Splintered time

Screening relied on identifying the earliest stages of disease: tuberculosis was the archetypal example – a small early lesion was easier to treat than a fulminating case in which the lungs were overwhelmed and the patient seriously ill. Clearly this strategy depended on a linear temporal model in which early small lesions grew larger and/or multiplied through the body. The post-war reconstruction of disease aetiology, however, undercut this step-wise picture of disease development, and redirected screening to new targets.

The celebrated Framingham study, started in 1948 to help identify the earliest precursors of heart disease, reported finding numerous potentially modifiable 'factors of risk' (Kannel *et al.* 1961). Detection of these risk factors re-ordered a medical framework which had assumed that degenerative processes, akin to the natural forces of decay, had underpinned chronic disease. The invention of risk factors – which began to have increasingly widespread use within medicine from the 1970s (see Figure 2) – at once affirmed the temporality of

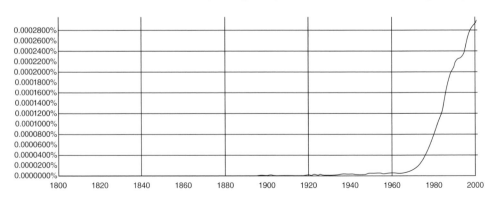

Figure 2 *'Risk factor' in Google Ngrams. The graph shows the frequency of keywords in a given year as a proportion of the total number of words in the database for that year (Michel et al. 2011)*

disease but also replaced its former linear spatialisation with a multi-dimensional one. Reliance of the screening project on identifying 'the' early manifestation of a disease was therefore unsustainable. As Arnott observed in 1954, the fact that effective prevention depended on knowledge of aetiology meant that 'At once, of course, one is up against the problem of multifactorial causation. There are few disease processes that can be assigned exclusively to a single cause' (1954: 887).

There had been occasional mention of the term 'multifactorial' before the 1950s but only in the context of the genetic determinants of disease. The post-war discovery of multiple risk factors and the rapid spread of 'multifactorial' as the aetiological descriptor for most, especially chronic, diseases undermined the linear developmental timeline on which screening was predicated (see Figure 3). If cardiovascular disease, for example, was 'caused' by high cholesterol, high blood pressure, obesity, smoking, lack of exercise, etc, how could screening hope to arrest its development? Indeed, even the earliest signs of disease were themselves further risk factors in the multidimensional array.

The initial reaction to the challenge of multifactorial aetiology was to extend screening to capture its proliferating targets. Multiphasic screening, which had earlier been promoted as a means of simultaneously addressing the timelines of multiple diseases, was adapted for the new task.

Multiphasic screening has been undergoing rapid changes in concept. Tests are becoming more sophisticated, quantitative and diagnostic; they are also becoming more risk factor oriented, and aimed at primary prevention. Most current programs include elements of both new concepts, and differ from earlier programs concerned only with presumptive identification of asymptomatic disease in presumably well persons (Thorner 1969: 1037).

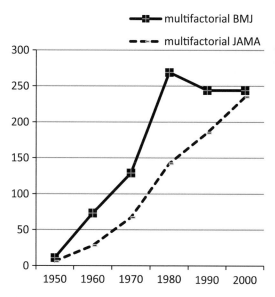

Figure 3 *'Multifactorial' Illustrative graph showing number of times indicated concept occurred in specific medical journals over 10 year periods. [BMJ = British Medical Journal; JAMA = Journal of the American Medical Association]*

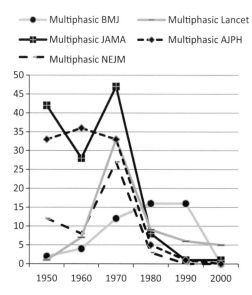

Figure 4 *'Multiphasic screening' Illustrative graph showing number of times indicated concept occurred in specific medical journals over 10 year periods. [BMJ = British Medical Journal; JAMA = Journal of the American Medical Association; Lancet; NEJM = New England Journal of Medicine; AJPH = American Journal of Public Health]*

In other words, instead of using screening to identify the earliest signs of disease (as in secondary prevention) it could be used to target risk factors and thereby prevent the disease even starting on its temporal trajectory.

Despite this promise, multiphasic screening as an approach to population surveillance proved short lived as it was rapidly overtaken by clinical strategies more compatible with a world of multiplying risk factors. Simultaneous identification of many latent diseases through multiphasic screening became obsolete once so many of these diseases were understood to rely on common risk factor pathways; by the 1980s multiphasic screening had fallen out of favour and by the 21st century had virtually disappeared (see Figure 4).

The subsequent history of screening was then marked by two divergent patterns. Some population screening survived but only for 'linear diseases' of which there were few, though even this remnant remained under increasing pressure. Otherwise, screening followed the risk factor as it proliferated and moved upstream, with less focus on disease timelines in a population and more on the temporal risk factor spaces of the individual patient. In effect, most of the post-war screening project was absorbed into routine clinical practice which increasingly turned to the identification and management of risk factors in individual patients in an opportunistic way.

The costs of screening

In the final two decades of the 20th century the post-war promise of population screening had been reduced to a handful of programmes suited to those diseases, especially cancers, with a seemingly uni-linear timeline or to maternity and child surveillance where future growth was at stake. But even these screening programmes came under challenge in the face of increasing awareness and attention to their potential costs and harms. At the centre of this critical new analysis of screening stood an emergent figure, that of the subjective and wilful patient.

It was known that some patients had blood pressures which seemed to vary day by day, hour by hour. These were labelled as 'labile hypertensives' (Locket 1955). But in 1984, in the context of understanding screening for high blood pressure, Kleinart and colleagues (1984) identified a new condition, 'white coat hypertension', which described the brief rise in blood pressure (presumably through patient anxiety) when it was being measured in the clinic. In other words, screening for hypertension could actually be creating the condition – or at least the appearance of the condition – it was designed to identify and manage. At the very least, this implied that many patients carried the label of (and took treatment for) hypertension when in fact their blood pressure was within normal limits. White coat hypertension illustrated two facets of the looming critique of screening. The first was the negative psychological reaction it could elicit in patients; the second were the more general harms which it could produce, particularly of over-treatment.

The idea that patients undergoing screening might have negative psychological reactions to the procedure became an important one during the 1980s. Clayman, for example, criticised the annual health check up in which 'Anxiety is created in the patient, and costly time is spent by the family physician providing reassurance for insignificant findings printed out in computer style and scrupulously sent to both family physician and patient' (Clayman 1980: 2067). In the 1980s increased anxiety was also reported in patients undergoing screening as varied as antenatal (Smithells 1980, Robinson *et al.* 1984), cervical screening (Wilkinson *et al.* 1990) and sickle cell disease (Consensus Conference 1987). This psychological response affected not only those found to be 'positive' but even those with normal results (Benfari *et al.* 1981, Burton *et al.* 1985).

A further facet of the patient's response to screening was the problem of uptake. Screening required the active participation of 'healthy' patients who were persuaded of the virtues of early detection across the disease's timeline. But a growing literature drew attention to the large proportion of eligible patients who failed to respond to the invitation to attend screening (see Figure 5). This 'failure' was yet another manifestation of the patient's psychological reaction to the procedure: as Merrick and colleagues (1985) noted with regard to breast cancer screening 'uptake of screening . . . seems likely also to depend on a woman's

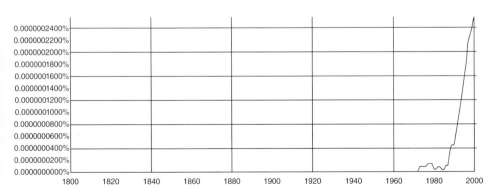

Figure 5 *'Uptake of Screening' in Google Ngrams. The graph shows the frequency of keywords in a given year as a proportion of the total number of words in the database for that year (Michel et al. 2011)*

underlying motivations and attitudes'. Screening uptake rates and means of increasing them therefore became a new focus for the screening agenda (Ross 1989, Thornton *et al.* 1995).

Unlike the traditional doctor-patient encounter where patients sought help by reporting their symptoms/illness, screening implied a different sort of contract; indeed, the consent implied by 'uptake' of the service could be absent. HIV antibody screening, for example, which could be conducted on blood taken for other purposes, became embroiled in ethical debates about consent, autonomy and potential harms (Bayer *et al.* 1986). Screening might provide benefit in terms of earlier diagnosis but it was clear that potential psychological and ethical harms were embedded in the very nature of the technology. Marteau (1990) concluded that 'all new screening programmes should include evaluation of the psychological impact of invitation and participation' (1990: 28).

While the psychological and ethical costs of participating in screening programmes received increasing attention, a further addition to the 'negative' side of the equation was emerging. All screening programmes were susceptible to 'misdiagnosis': sometimes patients were judged to be free of disease when in fact they had it (so-called false negatives) and sometimes patients were said to have the disease when in fact they did not (false positives). In the early years of screening the 'yield' of diseased patients was judged as the criterion of success but by the 1980s this figure was seen to consist of both true and false positives: what if most were the latter?

Figures for sensitivity and specificity had been used to characterise some laboratory tests since early in the century but were rarely calculated and reported for screening tests until the 1980s (though they had been recommended in Wilson and Jungner's (1968) 'Principles and practice of screening for disease'). Two further statistics appeared around this time, the test's positive predictive value (what proportion of patients identified as having disease actually did so), and negative predictive value (what proportion of patients identified as not having the disease actually did not). A frequent finding of these two statistics was the large number of patients who were misdiagnosed by screening tests. Irrespective of whether these misdiagnoses were false negatives or false positives they still carried costs for the patient: those with false negatives were falsely reassured while those who were false positive could undergo further investigation and even invasive treatments. Screening therefore became a trade-off between costs and benefits in which concern with uptake (by the non-adherent patient) began to be replaced by a new discourse on informed choice in which the individual patient had to decide whether to attend, once appraised of all the evidence. Meta-analyses of breast cancer trials, for example, estimated that for every one women who benefited from screening (in terms of her life being saved) a further ten women underwent the same treatments but unnecessarily (Gøtzsche and Nielsen 2010). Women could therefore be asked to add their personal values to the cost-benefit equation before reaching an individual decision on whether the screening was likely to be advantageous or harmful (McPherson 2010).

In 1974 Ingelfinger critically observed that the screening bandwagon seemed unstoppable as even sceptics had to concede that 'screening programs will be used whether or not any evidence is available that they improve the health of the people' (Ingelfinger 1974: 99–100). Just over a decade later a new more cautious assessment had emerged. In a review of breast cancer screening in 1988, for example, Eddy and his colleagues tried to balance the various costs and benefits of screening according to contemporary evidence. The actual 'disease' was not their central concern nor the characteristics of its earliest manifestations; instead they placed survival benefit in a matrix of anxiety, inconvenience, false sense of security, distress, disfigurement and disability. This calculus was to be frequently reworked in later years and with it came the increasing psychologisation of patients as their reactions, subjectivities and choices were dissected, calibrated and summed. The term 'harms of screening'

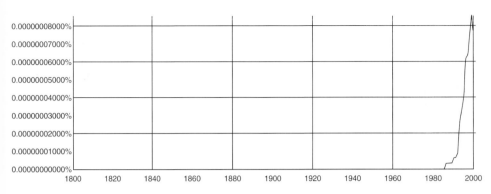

Figure 6 *'Harms of screening' in Google Ngrams. The graph shows the frequency of keywords in a given year as a proportion of the total number of words in the database for that year (Michel et al. 2011)*

was totally absent in the medical literature up until the 1990s; since then it can be found with increasing frequency (see Figure 6).

Time and subjectivity

Screening is a 20th century phenomenon. The word itself has its origins in both the X-ray screen and the public health mesh which separated flies from humans and solids from smaller particles. Since then screening has been both dependent on and reinforced by transformations in clinical practice. The first of these is the identification of a timeline for diseases, that they have latent, early and late manifestations, such that intervention towards the beginning of this natural history can change an otherwise predestined outcome. This principle can also be applied to apparently 'normal' populations (which, after application of the screening programme, are invariably no longer normal). These two constructs informed a new form of Surveillance Medicine which began to replace Pathological Medicine during the late 20th century (Armstrong 1995).

When screening programmes first appeared, they targeted diseases which threatened others. This principle was applied during World War II to embrace all those diseases which might affect a community at war such as tuberculosis, venereal disease and mental disease. Prior to the war, screening had also been applied to the health of school-children on the basis that abnormalities in the child could affect later adulthood. It was this intra-individual threat that underpinned post-war initiatives as screening technologies were applied to the growing numbers of diseases contained within the chronic disease classification which, like the problem of the child in the inter-war years, was a threat to the future of the individual rather than of others. The labelling of cancer, cardiovascular disease, diabetes, rheumatic fever, etc, as chronic diseases opened up new targets for screening programmes.

Screening implied a different type of doctor-patient encounter. Clinical practice at the start of the 20th century involved patients reporting their symptoms to doctors who then, after clinical examination and appropriate investigations, made a diagnosis. The idea of population screening changed that relationship: it was the doctor who sought out the asymptomatic patient who would be unaware of the potential diseases they carried. The focus was not therefore the consulting patient but the non-consulting one, the anonymous person in the population, outside of medical care. Use of the term 'case finding' captured something of this search for unknown disease in the population (though all diagnosis was a sort of case finding). Yet these hidden cases did not have to be identified through 'mass' population screening. The advent of multifactorial aetiology demanded new strategies for early risk factor/disease identification and intervention. The problem, to be sure, was located in the population but rising use of healthcare meant that most of the population could be surveyed when they consulted on other matters. A number of new tactics therefore emerged to replace population screening: periodic examinations, health checks, medical check-ups, risk-profiling, opportunistic screening, etc, together with recruitment of the patient to their own risk factor management. All these approaches involved not only a search for early manifestations of disease in asymptomatic patients but also for even earlier threats. In this way screening, which had originated as a population-wide strategy, moved to the centre of individual clinical practice, more local, less formal, more penetrating, and less resistible.

The absorption of screening techniques into routine risk factor medicine and the contemporary identification of immanent harms of screening programmes meant that the post-war dream of a surveillance society in which mass populations were processed through screening programmes to identify early disease proved transitory. What remains of population screening stands under threat, defended by those such as lay groups and lobbyists who continue to promote the post-war belief in the inherent virtues of the prevention/screening paradigm. When the US Preventive Services Task Force, for example, recommended that women aged 40–49 should make 'individual decisions' about whether to undergo breast cancer screening given that harms might outweigh benefits, it was met by such fierce opposition from various lay and professional interest groups that the debate was characterised as 'the mammographic wars' (Quanstrum and Hayward 2010). The core preventive idea that inspired the screening movement in the 20th century, that disease was better detected early, clearly retains much of its potency for the many lay groups and, indeed, for the many clinical constituencies which are actively involved in delivering screening programmes. Yet the construction of a countervailing thesis (by epidemiologists, psychologists, ethicists and other clinicians) of harms and costs has now established a significant barrier to the introduction of future population screening, as well as forged a critique which is likely to continue to challenge existing programmes. The case for screening was often promoted through the iconic voice of the individual patient whose life had been 'saved'; nowadays identifying that fortunate patient in the midst of all the false positive cases has become an all but impossible task.

One of the many challenges that population screening faced in the closing decades of the 20th century was its engagement with the ethical and psychological patient. This figure was new. In part it was a shape illuminated by the sharp light of screening technologies; but it was also the analysis of the harms of screening over the last three decades which served to construct and affirm the identity of the subjective autonomous patient, not least from sociological writings critical of the objectifying nature of screening procedures (McKie 1995). Screening, as Howson (1999) argued, 'was embedded in a moral framework of self responsibility and social obligation' (1999: 401). In effect, patients' negative psychological reactions to screening both constrained the uncritical expansion of screening but also provided a point of articulation for the increasingly voluble research literature which showed again and again that patients were more than the passive recipients of medical procedures (Marteau et al. 1993, Sutton et al. 1995, Neher 1999, Consedine et al. 2004, Brunton et al. 2005). Debates at the interface between screening and patient autonomy and integrity have therefore provided an important medium through which that identity could be rehearsed and stabilised.

The new figure of the patient which materialised from the screening project was invested with time. Screening itself was a temporal project as were the illnesses it targeted. In the early years of screening disease timelines criss-crossed populations but in the immediate post-war years the timelines shifted from populations to individuals. The degenerative processes of chronic illness mapped out the temporal space of individuality – a configuration which informed what is now referred to as a 'life-course' perspective. The temporal space of the individual then began to fragment. Multi-factorial risk factor aetiology located illness in a multidimensional space (itself a construct of the second half of the 20th century) undermining the solitary disease trajectory which had justified the earlier population screening regime. The idea of causation itself contained a temporal ordering whereby an earlier event determined a later one. The emergence of multifactorial aetiology further emphasised this temporality of illness (and also undermines the possibility of identifying the basis of this change in causal frameworks as the explanation of the explanatory model is contained within itself). The fusion of screening technologies and individual practice produced more opportunistic surveillance and with it a multidimensional biographical space enveloping each separate patient. This process was reinforced by the vestiges of the population screening project which, in the face of psychological, ethical and medical challenges, moved the focus of the medical gaze towards the subjective and autonomous patient who was a model of individual decision-making and informed choice.

Acknowledgements

I would like to thank the Monograph Editors, Natalie Armstrong and Helen Eborall, and the Monograph Series Editor, Hannah Bradby, for helpful comments and suggestions on an earlier draft.

References

AJPH Editorial (1932) Child hygiene: Tuberculosis in childhood, *American Journal of Public Health*, 22, 1309–1312.

Armstrong, D. (1995) The rise of Surveillance Medicine, *Sociology of Health and Illness*, 17, 393–404.

Arnott, W.M. (1954) The changing aetiology of heart disease, *British Medical Journal*, 2, 887–91.

Bayer, R., Levine, C. and Wolf, S.M. (1966) HIV antibody screening: an ethical framework for evaluating proposed programs, *Journal of the American Medical Association*, 256, 1768–74.

Benfari, R.C., Eaker, E., McIntyre, K. and Paul, O. (1981) Risk factor screening and intervention: a psychological / behavioral cost or a benefit? *Control Clinical Trials*, 2, 3–14.

Bentley, F.J. and Leitner, Z.A. (1940) Mass radiography, *British Medical Journal*, 1, 879–83.

Brunton, M., Jordan, C. and Campbell, I. (2005) Anxiety before, during, and after participation in a population-based screening mammography programme in Waikato Province, *New Zealand, New Zealand Medical Journal*, 118, 1299.

Burton, B.K., Dillard, R.G. and Clark, E.N. (1985) Maternal serum alpha-fetoprotein screening: the effect of participation on anxiety and attitude toward pregnancy in women with normal results, *American Journal of Obstetrics and Gynaecology*, 152, 540–3.

Buck, C.E. (1925) School health examinations, *American Journal of Public Health*, 15, 972–7.

Capon, N.B. (1950) Development and behaviour of children, *British Medical Journal*, 1, 859–69.

Carroll, H.J. (1976) Preparing for screening for hypertension in the community, *Bulletin of the New York Academy of Medicine*, 52, 646–7.

Champion, M.E. (1925) Should the health examination be a screening or a diagnosis? *American Journal of Public Health*, 15, 1083–5.

Chapman, A.L. (1949) The concept of multiphasic screening, *Public Health Reports*, 64, 1311–4.

Ciocco, A. (1945) Physical growth in childhood and military fitness, *American Journal of Public Health*, 35, 927–33.

Clayman, C.B. (1980) Mass screening: is it cost-effective? *Journal of the American Medical Association*, 243, 2067–8.

Conference Report (1931) Prevention of tuberculosis, *British Medical Journal*, 2, 28–9.

Consedine, N.S., Magai, C., Krivoshekova, Y.S., Ryzewicz, L. and Neugut, A.I. (2004) Fear, anxiety, worry, and breast cancer screening behavior: a critical review, *Cancer Epidemiology, Biomarkers and Prevention*, 13, 501–10.

Consensus Conference (1987) Anxiety is a risk of screening: Newborn Screening for sickle cell disease and other haemoglobinopathies, *Journal of the American Medical Association*, 258, 1205–9.

Cooper, E.L. (1940) Pulmonary tuberculosis in recruits. Experiences in a survey by the microradiographic method, *British Medical Journal*, 2, 245–8.

Dale, H. (1932) Therapeutic problems of the future, *British Medical Journal*, 2, 1151–2.

Deibert, A.V. (1948) Recent developments in cancer control, *American Journal of Public Health*, 38, 191–201.

Dugan, S.V. (1932) Public Health Administration: Short schools for milk control officials, *American Journal of Public Health*, 22, 1287–90.

Dunbar, F. (1945) Public health aspects of psychosomatic problems, *American Journal of Public Health*, 35, 117–22.

Eddy, D.M., Hasselblad, V, McGivney, W. and Hendee, W. (1988) The Value of Mammography Screening in Women Under Age 50 Years, *Journal of the American Medical Association*, 259, 1512–9.

Enos, W.F., Holmes, R.H. and Beyer, J. (1953) Coronary heart disease among United States soldiers killed in action in Korea, *Journal of the American Medical Association*, 152, 1090–3.

Freemont-Smith, M. (1953) Periodic examination of supposedly well persons, *New England Journal of Medicine*, 248, 170–3.

Gøtzsche, P.C. and Nielsen, M. (2010) Screening for breast cancer with mammography, *Cochrane Database Systematic Review*, 340:c3106 doi: 10.1136/bmj.c3106.

Halverson, W.L., Breslow, L. and Merrill, M.H. (1949) The Chronic Disease Study of the California Department of Public Health, *American Journal of Public Health*, 39, 593–7.

Hetherington, H.W., McPhedran, F.M., Landis, H.R.M. and Opie, E.L. (1931) Tuberculosis in medical and college students, *Archives of Internal Medicine*, 48, 734–63.

Holmes, E.M., Bowden, P.W. and Warner, G.W. (1954) Multiphasic Screening: Evaluation as tool in chronic disease control program, *Southern Medical Journal*, 47, 117–182.

Howson, A. (1999) Cervical screening, compliance and moral obligation, *Sociology of Health and Illness*, 21, 401–25.

Hubbard, J.P. (1957) *Early Detection and Prevention of Disease*. New York: McGraw-Hill.

Ingefinger, F.J. (1974) Multiphasic screening. In Inglefinger, F.J., Ebert, R.V., Finland, M. and Relman, A.S. (eds). *Controversy in Internal Medicine II*. Philadelphia: WB Saunders.

JAMA Editorial (1950) Chronic illness, *Journal of the American Medical Association*, 144, 466.

JAMA Editorial (1950) Discovering unsuspected diabetes, *Journal of the American Medical Association*, 144, 468–9.

James, G. (1955) Screening for heart disease, *Journal of Chronic Diseases*, 2, 440–9.

Jones, H.W. and Cameron, W.R. (1947) Case-finding factors in cancer detection centres, *Journal of the American Medical Association*, 135, 964–7.

Kannel, W.B., Dawber, T.R., Kagan, A., Revotskie, N. and Stokes, J. (1961) Factors of risk in the development of coronary heart disease–six year follow-up experience: The Framingham Study, *Annals of Internal Medicine*, 55, 33–50.

Kleinert, H.D., Harshfield, G.A., Pickering, T.G, Devereux, R.B., Sullivan, P.A., Marion, R.M., Mallory, W.K. and Laragh, J.H. (1984) What is the value of home blood pressure measurement in patients with mild hypertension? *Hypertension*, 6, 574–8.

Lancet Editorial (1899) The sewage-fed Orwell Estuary, *Lancet*, 154, 39–40.

Lang, F.R. (1941) What the Navy is doing to protect its personnel against venereal disease, *American Journal of Public Health*, 31, 1032–9.

Lawson, D. and Crombie, R.H. (1903) Roentgen rays in the diagnosis of lung disease, *Lancet*, 162, 212–4.

Levin, M. (1951) Detection of chronic disease, *Journal of the American Medical Association*, 146, 1397–1401.

Locket, S. (1955) Oral Preparations of Rauwolfia Serpentina in Treatment of Essential Hypertension, *British Medical Journal*, 1, 809.

Long, E.R. and Lew, E.A. (1945) Tuberculosis in the Armed Forces, *American Journal of Public Health*, 35, 469–79.

Marteau, T.M. (1990) Reducing the psychological costs, *British Medical Journal*, 301, 26–8.

Marteau, T.M., Kidd, J., Michie, S., Cook, R., Johnston, M. and Shaw, R.W. (1993) Anxiety, knowledge and satisfaction in women receiving false positive results on routine prenatal screening: a randomized controlled trial, *Journal of Psychosomatic Obstetrics and Gynecology*, 14, 185–96.

McKie, L. (1995) The art of surveillance or reasonable prevention? The case of cervical screening, *Sociology of Health and Illness*, 17, 441–57.

McPherson, K. (2010) Screening for breast cancer – balancing the debate, *British Medical Journal*, 340:c3106.

Merrick, M.V., Eastwood, M.A. and Ford, M.J. (1985) Is bile acid malabsorption underdiagnosed? An evaluation of accuracy of diagnosis by measurement of SeHCAT retention, *British Medical Journal*, 290, 665.

Michel, J.-B., Shen, Y.K., Aiden, A.P., Veres, A., Gray, M.K., The Google Books Team, Pickett, J.P., Hoiberg, D., Clancy, D., Norvig, P., Orwant, J., Pinker, S., Nowak, M.A. and Aiden, E.L. (2011) Quantitative Analysis of Culture Using Millions of Digitized Books, *Science*, 14 January 2011: 176–82.

Neher, J.O. (1999) Reducing patient anxiety about positive screening tests, *American Family Physician*, 59, 2714–7.

Oak, L. (1942) The Massachusetts Vision Test: An improved method for school vision testing, *American Journal of Public Health*, 32, 1105–9.

Papanicolaou, G.N. (1948) The cell smear method of diagnosing cancer, *American Journal of Public Health*, 38, 202–5.

Papanicolaou, G.N. and Traut, H.F. (1943) *The diagnosis of uterine cancer by the vaginal smear*. New York: Commonwealth Fund.

Perrott, G.S. (1944) Content and administration of a medical care program: Training of personnel and research, *American Journal of Public Health*, 34, 1244–51.

Perrott, G.S. (1945) A comprehensive training program for public health personnel, *American Journal of Public Health*, 35, 1155–62.

Quanstrum, K.H. and Hayward, R.A. (2010) Lessons from the Mammography Wars, *New England Journal of Medicine*, 363, 1076–9.

Robinson, G.C. (1941) Health problems in national defense, *American Journal of Public Health*, 31, 969–976.

Robinson, J.O., Hibbard, B.M. and Laurence, K.M.J. (1984) Anxiety during a crisis: emotional effects of screening for neural tube defects, *Psychosomatic Research*, 28, 163–9.

Ross, S.K. (1989) Cervical cytology screening and government policy, *British Medical Journal*, 299, 101 doi:10.1136/bmj.299.6691.101.

Rowntree, L.G. (1944) National program for physical fitness revealed and developed on the basis of 13,000 physical examinations of selective service registrants, *Journal of the American Medical Association*, 125, 821–7.

Schenthal, J.E. (1960) Multiphasic screening of the well patient: twelve-year experience of the Tulane University Cancer Detection Clinic, *Journal of the American Medical Association*, 172, 1–4.

Shepard, W.P., Atwater, R.M., Anderson, G.W., Bauer, W.W., Defries, R.D., Godfrey, E.S., McIver, P., Ramsey, G.H., Reed, L.J., Smillie, W.G., Stebbins, E.L., Tarbett, R.E., Turner, C.E., Wilson, C.C., Carey, E.J., Guthrie, W.G., Kleinschmidt, E.E., Mitchell, H.H., Sellery, C.M. and Wheatley,

G.M. (1944) Report of the Committee on Professional Education, *American Journal of Public Health*, 34, 977–3.

Sisson, J.H. (1957) Periodic examination of well patients, *Medical Clinics of North America*, 41, 1439–49.

Smithells, R.W. (1980) AFP screening and maternal anxiety, *Lancet*, 1, 772–3.

Soper, G.A. (1914) Rational basis for the sanitation of rivers and harbours, *American Journal of Public Health*, 4, 1089–92.

Sutton, S., Saidi, G., Bickler, G. and Hunter, J. (1995) Does routine screening for breast cancer raise anxiety? Results from a three wave prospective study in England, *Journal of Epidemiology and Community Health*, 49, 413–8.

Thorner, R.M. (1969) Whither Multiphasic Screening? *New England Journal of Medicine*, 280, 1037–42.

Thornton, J.G., Hewison, J., Lilford, R.J. and Vail, A. (1995) A randomised trial of three methods of giving information about prenatal testing, *British Medical Journal*, 311, 1127.

Wakefield, P. (1930) Children's tuberculosis program in Massachusetts, *New England Journal of Medicine*, 203, 168–172.

Webb, E.L. and Sellers, T.F. (1943) Four years' use of the Kahn Presumptive Test as a screening agency in the serology of syphilis, *American Journal of Public Health*, 33, 537–40.

Wilkerson, H.L.C. and Ford, M.J. (1949) Diabetes control in a local Health Department, *American Journal of Public Health*, 39, 607–13.

Wilkerson, H.L.C., Cohen, A.S. and Kenedjian, B.G. (1955) Screening for diabetes, *Journal of Chronic Disease*, 2, 464–76.

Wilkinson, C., Jones, J.M. and McBride, J. (1990) Anxiety caused by abnormal result of cervical smear test: a controlled trial, *British Medical Journal*, 300, 440.

Wilson, C.C. (1946) A new statement of school health policies, *American Journal of Public Health*, 36, 58–60.

Wilson, J.M.G. and Jungner, G. (1968) Principles and practice of screening for disease, *WHO Chronicle*, 22, 473: Public Health Papers No.34.

3

The experience of risk as 'measured vulnerability': health screening and lay uses of numerical risk

Chris Gillespie

Introduction

Health risk has become ubiquitous in today's society. Media reports of elevated risk occur regularly, including countless special reports on new strategies for reducing risk and the development of numerous screening programs aimed at identifying those who are at risk (Brown *et al*. 1996). These reports range from the identification of behavioural traits that should be modified to the introduction of specific foods into one's diet (Nerlich and Koteyko 2008). Rosenberg (2009) refers to this contemporary climate as one of 'ambient risk'. It seems as though there is no getting away from risk, or at least there's no getting away from being bombarded with information about health risk.

The identification of risk is accomplished through medical and public health profession-als that have come to increasingly rely upon health screening in everyday practice. How risk is understood by lay persons influences the way they experience having characteristics that increase their risk for serious health conditions (Garrety 1998, Nettleton *et al*. 2005). However, statistical risk is widely misunderstood by lay persons, fuelled by media reporting and representations of risk, and often misapplied by health professionals (Kabat 2008, Brown *et al*. 1996, Nelkin 1989, Lidskog 1996).

While numbers might be the ultimate abstractions, they have been ascribed the status of reliability, and of certainty (Woodward 1999). Risk is a measure of the probability of a future event. Rather than recognising that averages are based upon aggregate populations, they are viewed as hard realities, or as ideals to which individuals should aspire. Lay under-standings of risk differ considerably from expert interpretations, as lay persons typically react with greater alarm (Siegrist *et al*. 2007) or with a sense of fatalism (Keeley *et al*. 2009). In this essay, lay meanings of numerical measures of risk will be explored in order to deter-mine the extent to which statistics become reified through individual experience.

Conceptualising risk

The rise of the use of risk in health monitoring has been attributed to the expansion of surveillance medicine (Armstrong 1995). Much of the rise of surveillance medicine can be attributed to the development of the risk factor, and the use of risk factors in monitoring health at both the population and individual level (Aronowitz 1998). Risk factors are

The Sociology of Medical Screening, First Edition. Edited by Natalie Armstrong and Helen Eborall.
Chapters © 2012 The Authors. Book Compilation © 2012 Foundation for the Sociology of Health
& Illness / Blackwell Publishing Ltd. Published 2012 by Blackwell Publishing Ltd.

statistical measures of individual characteristics that increase the probability of adverse health events. Risk is employed in a manner that expands medical influence through the incorporation of an ever-increasing range of health-related phenomena (Conrad 2007). A hallmark of contemporary medical practice is the treatment of risk factors, or the treatment of 'conditions' that have been identified as contributing to ill health, but that do not presently produce suffering (Armstrong 1995, Greaves 2000). Risk becomes medicalised as it becomes a condition that is treated in itself (Aronowitz 2009, Arnst 1999). While risk is not the presence of disease, it is often treated through medical means, including medication, behaviour modification, and surgical intervention.

There is an important distinction between thinking of risk as a statistical category, as an objective condition, or as a social condition of compromised health status. It is this function of risk as a social condition that is the focus of this research. Conceptualising risk for this purpose is a challenging task. My intent is to use the experiences of those who are at risk as the basis for a more refined conceptualisation of risk, one rooted in the social experiences of those who are determined to be at risk. Those who find themselves 'at risk' derive unique meaning from the term. This conceptual complexity is a fundamental aspect of what I am attempting to address in this research.

The experience of illness framework
As more aspects of everyday life are pathologised, risk becomes a central component in how people manage their health, and their lives. One of the arguments of this research is that as risk becomes a condition to be treated in itself, it has come to be viewed as an illness. And, as such, it has begun to be experienced as an illness.

The study of the illness experience has generated conceptual understandings of being ill as biographical disruption (Bury 1982, 1991), as loss of self (Charmaz 1983, 1987), or as narrative reconstruction (Williams 2000). These concepts emerge from accounts of those who are ill in order to determine the character of the experience of illness.

Studying the experiences of those designated as being at increased health risk allows for greater understanding of the meanings people attach to individual health status and of the impact this perceived status has on their everyday, lived-realities. This approach makes possible the emergence of an 'insider's perspective' on being at risk, allowing the experiences, meanings, and social interactions of those designated as such to inform the elaboration of the experience of risk, rather than merely assigning meaning deductively (Schneider and Conrad, 1983).

This research was designed to specifically target the experience of risk through the study of those who have been designated as being at risk for a serious health condition. The meanings people attach to health risk in their lives, as well as their strategies for managing risk are explored. Additionally, an analysis of the experience of risk has the capacity for pointing towards an appropriate sociological characterisation of this experience and of a conceptualisation of health risk, relative to health and illness.

Methodology

In order to grasp the experience of living with health risk I chose to compare two cases in which people were designated as being at increased risk of a serious health condition. In each case, risk was measured numerically, through routine health screening.

The first case that was examined included men and women with elevated blood cholesterol levels. High cholesterol (hypercholesterolemia) has been linked to an increased risk of coronary heart disease and stroke. Along with hypertension and obesity, high cholesterol is considered a significant risk factor for heart disease, and has been highly publicised in the media as a condition which should be monitored by adults throughout the developed world.

The US Centers for Disease Control and Prevention estimate that over 16 per cent of adults in the US have cholesterol levels which place them at high risk for coronary heart disease (240+ mg/dL), and 50 per cent of adults have levels above 200, considered to be at elevated risk. The mean serum cholesterol level for all US adults is 203 (NCHS 2009).

The second case that was examined included men with an elevated prostate-specific antigen level (PSA) as indicated by a PSA test. The PSA test is used as a screening tool in the diagnosis of prostate cancer. Elevated levels of PSA in a man's blood may indicate the presence of prostate cancer, which can be confirmed through prostate biopsy. The American Cancer Society recommends that men over the age of 50 receive yearly screening for prostate cancer using both Digital Rectal Exams and PSA tests as diagnostic tools. Males with elevated PSA levels are considered to be at increased risk of the presence of prostate cancer.

Men with a PSA level of 10 ng/mL or higher are considered to be at increased risk of prostate cancer. Approximately 67 per cent of men in the US with PSA levels above this threshold are later diagnosed with prostate cancer (Catalona 1992). While there is no consensus as to what constitutes a normal PSA level (some, including the US National Cancer Society, consider levels below 4.0 ng/mL to be normal, while others, such as the American Urological Association, use a more stringent level of 2.5 ng/mL), it is estimated that among those with levels between 4 and 10 ng/mL, 25 per cent result in biopsy-proven prostate cancer (Eastham *et al*. 2003). Therefore, the 4–10 PSA range is considered that of moderate risk.

These cases are similar in that they both involve screening for early detection of underlying conditions whereby risk is assigned through numerical measures. Both cases have thresholds above which a person is considered to be at risk. People with a total blood cholesterol level of 240 mg/dL or greater are considered to be at risk (*high*) for coronary heart disease. However, those whose cholesterol level falls within the 200–239 range are considered to have an *elevated* cholesterol level and are often considered to be at increased risk of heart disease as well. A total cholesterol level of less than 200 is considered to be desirable (NCEP 2001).

Both cases include blood tests, which are routine parts of regular health exams in the US. Also, both cholesterol levels and PSA levels are not considered, of themselves, to be discreet health conditions. In other words, abnormal results do not indicate ill health in a clinical sense, and have no associated symptoms. However, while both cases are considered risk factors for serious health conditions, they each serve as risk factors in different ways and each has a distinct history that contributes to how they function as a risk factor.

The major difference in the case of PSA is that while cholesterol levels are seen as a contributing factor to heart disease, PSA levels are simply an indicator of the possible existence of prostate cancer. While elevated PSA levels increase a person's risk of prostate cancer, reducing those levels will not have any impact on the presence or absence of prostate cancer. PSA does not contribute to the development of cancer in any way, with increased levels merely indicating the possible presence of cancer, suggesting the appropriateness of further confirmatory testing through biopsy.

The cases of elevated cholesterol and elevated PSA levels act as risk factors because neither provides a definitive diagnosis of coronary heart disease or of prostate cancer, respectively. They are both indirect measures of disease. Elevated cholesterol levels represent a greater likelihood of the development of disease at some future point, while elevated

PSA levels indicate an increased likelihood of the current presence of disease. As indirect measures, however, elevated cholesterol and PSA levels leave the individual in a state of being at risk for something which is either yet to develop or is yet to be discovered. This space of medical uncertainty allows for the study of the experience of being at risk.

The study included interviews with 21 people who had elevated cholesterol levels, and 21 men with elevated PSA levels. Those with elevated cholesterol levels ranged in age from 26 to 75, with a median age of 45. Eleven of these participants were male (52%), while the other ten were female (48%). However, as prostate cancer only affects men, participants with elevated PSA levels were exclusively male. Men in this case ranged in age from 50 to 79 years of age, with a median age of 60. This older cohort is due to current recommendations to begin PSA screening at age 50.

The analysis of data consisted of coding interview transcripts, making notes of themes that emerged from the data and drawing conclusions that led to a conceptualisation of the risk experience for those who participated in the study. As this study included two distinct cases, it was useful to analyse each case separately, looking for themes that were particular to each case, then making comparisons across cases in order to develop a general framework of the experience of being at risk.

The risk experience

> I think I'd always thought of myself as an absolutely healthy person and no particular problems whatsoever, and having this sudden abnormality was sort of the first – the first stone dropped in the pond, so to speak (Robert).

Robert's statement indicates that being designated as being at increased risk can be the beginning of an experience that revolves around a compromised health status. Note that I am careful not to characterise this experience as one of compromised health, but rather of compromised status as a healthy person. Robert's inability to continue to think of himself as a healthy person is indicative of the experience of many of those I spoke with.

Robert's identification of this initial discovery as the 'first stone' astutely recognises that it is just the beginning of an experience that will often include the dropping of other stones in the future. Also, the imagery of a stone dropping in a pond vividly alludes to how the designation of risk causes ripples that extend outward, impacting on other aspects of a person's social world.

The application of risk numbers yielded a pervasive sense of impending ill health that many participants embodied in a way that made a reconstruction of identity necessary. Reorganising identity and altering conceptualisations of personal health leads to uncertainty about current health status as well as future prospects for health. Ultimately, being at risk led to altered health identities and a sense of what I term 'measured vulnerability'.

Altered health status

Being at risk altered respondents' perceptions of their health. Jonathan, thinking back to when he was diagnosed with elevated cholesterol, said, 'I was in perfect health until about a year and a half ago'. For Jonathan, being designated as at risk, as a result of his cholesterol levels, represented a change in his health status.

Being at risk was discrediting to a healthy identity, having the effect of spoiling one's identity (Goffman 1963). Meyers (2003) notes that when people who are at risk interact with others, 'they are not just presenting an evaluation of probabilities and dangers, they are representing and defending versions of themselves' (2003: 215). Successfully managing risk by reducing abnormal cholesterol or PSA levels was considered to be an accomplishment that would make respondents feel better about themselves, reducing the perceived stigma that resulted from their risk status.

Indicator of advancing age
Many respondents interpreted being at risk as an indication of advancing age. Those with elevated cholesterol levels tended to take their risk status as a sign that they were ageing prematurely. At 33, Ken felt as though his elevated cholesterol was something that suggested a decline in his health. Referring to his cholesterol, Ken said, 'I guess similar to many areas of ill health, it's something that tends to get worse as you get older unless you take drastic measures'. This sense of premature ageing was often concerning for respondents.

Those with elevated PSA levels, on the other hand, interpreted their risk status as something that was a natural part of ageing. Rising PSA levels were interpreted merely as part of a general deterioration of the body, something they expected to occur as they aged. Jared referred to his PSA level as 'Middle-age stuff, you know, memory issues, sometimes, energy issues, and this prostate . . .'

Regardless of whether advancing age as a result of increased risk was interpreted as premature, or as something more natural, being at risk was interpreted by respondents as evidence that they were getting older. Equating risk with age indicates that respondents were facing mortality as a result of having been designated as being at risk. In Jared's words, 'It certainly means the clock is ticking'.

Pervasiveness of risk
The most common characterisation of the saliency of being at risk for respondents was that it was always in the back of their minds. While not continually conscious of one's risk status, respondents felt, nonetheless, as though it was something that was always there. Matt said, 'In the back of your mind it's sort of something that's there.' Also, Charles said, 'It's there somewhere back here. You know?'

The pervasiveness of having, in the back of your mind, a sense that your health has been compromised was an important element of the risk experience for respondents. Respondents cited meals, taking medication or supplements, and follow-up screenings as times when their risk status became more salient (Paterson 2001).

When I asked Ken when he thought about his elevated cholesterol levels, he said, 'Every time I sit down to a meal now, I think I have high cholesterol'. The association between cholesterol and food led respondents to think about their risk status at times when food was present.

Medication serves as a reminder to people that they have a health condition that needs attention (Conrad 1985). Taking medication or using natural supplements also served as triggers that reminded respondents of their elevated cholesterol or PSA levels (Pound *et al.* 2005). Brenda said, 'The medication reminds you a little bit'. Medication and supplements were daily reminders, or at least regular reminders, that became part of respondents' routines.

The most critical reminders of risk, the events that triggered the most salient response to risk, were screening tests. This was primarily a factor for those with elevated PSA levels. Matt's PSA had remained steady for a number of years and at the time of our interview he was receiving PSA tests annually. Matt said, 'At the time that I was visiting this urologist every six months; it was probably way in my mind more. Because I had these doctor appointments'. Frequent medical contact kept risk salient for respondents (see Fowler 2006).

Between screenings, respondents indicated that their risk status would typically recede to the backs of their minds. Charles noted, 'I didn't think too much about it until it came up on the six months and the time I had the blood test. And then once I had the . . . blood test and waiting for the results I think about it everyday'. The period between receiving the PSA test and receiving the results was a very anxious time for many respondents, and being at risk was much more pervasive in their immediate thoughts during those times.

Identity and embodiment
The lack of symptoms associated with elevated cholesterol or PSA levels, as well as with many other risk factors, seemed to intensify the pervasiveness of respondents' risk status as they were unable to determine their individual risk without undergoing additional screening tests. The experience of risk is one in which people are no longer able to rely on self-monitoring of health through physical cues, or symptoms, that would indicate either the deterioration or improvement of health. The risk experience leads to a compromised ability to trust one's body to communicate health status. As Armstrong (1995) writes, 'It is no longer the symptom or sign pointing tantalizingly at the hidden pathological truth of disease, but the risk factor opening up a space of future illness potential' (1995: 400).

Those with elevated PSA levels internalised the presence of cancer within their bodies. Archie said, 'What was not detectable in 2006 could've raised its ugly head in 2007, and it didn't'. A negative prostate biopsy did not indicate to Archie that he was cancer-free, just that it was possible that the cancer had not shown itself yet. This is similar to the conceptualisation of cancer as an invasion of the body (Weiss 1997). Those with elevated PSA levels often acted as though they had prostate cancer, regardless of a lack of diagnosis.

Brian said that he was relieved when his prostate biopsies would come back negative for cancer, but noted that he was often surprised because he was convinced that cancer existed and that it was just a matter of time until it was discovered. He said, 'I honestly figure I'm going to have it at some point'. Later in the interview, Brian was very specific in saying, 'Since April 12th, 1999 I've felt it's coming'. Since the date of Brian's first biopsy, he felt prostate cancer was inevitable.

While the embodiment of cancer was specific to those with elevated PSA levels, respondents from both cases embodied their risk status not in terms of statistical probability, as is suggested by risk, but as potential. For those with elevated cholesterol levels, this embodiment was most commonly reflected metaphorically through descriptions of the self as a 'ticking time bomb'.

Referring to her cholesterol levels and the potential for heart disease, Janet said, 'I'm a walking time bomb . . . I could explode!' Others used similar remarks, with Sarah saying, 'I'm kind of a ticking time bomb right now'. Gene also explained it as follows:

> It's sort of like – it's a combination between a trip wire booby trap and a time bomb . . . A trip wire booby trap but if you don't trip the wire, it doesn't go off. So, if you watch your cholesterol, then you should be fine. However, there's the time bomb part . . . that part you can't do anything about.

Thinking of elevated cholesterol as something within the body that could explode was also related to a sense of cholesterol leading to a heart attack.

The embodiment of risk made it difficult for respondents to maintain an identity as a healthy person. The presence of risk meant respondents were no longer able to act as though they would have a healthy life, but that it was necessary to think of their lives as limited, or as finite. Many participants indicated that being at risk meant they were no longer immortal, or that they were no longer able to perceive themselves as invincible.

Respondents used such terms as 'invincible', 'indestructible', 'immortal', or 'superman' to refer to their identities prior to the designation of risk, but indicated that they were no longer able to think of themselves in such terms. The experience of risk led respondents to feel vulnerable and necessitated a revision of their identity in order to accommodate a susceptibility to potential disease. A designation of risk removed a perceived buffer between health and illness. Respondents were not able to assume that they were exempt from the possibility of chronic illness due to their age, lack of symptoms, or sense of 'invincibility'. Being at risk pushed them to the brink of illness, a place where they felt vulnerable.

While epidemiologists use risk factors to calculate health risk, respondents thought of factors such as age, family history, and risk numbers as possible buffers to ill health. This signifies a conceptualisation in which there is a space between health and illness. This space represents a cushion, or protective buffer, that must be breached prior to the onset of illness.

The presence of risk factors for disease weakened this buffer, bringing them closer to illness. Therefore, as one ages, the buffer is weakened. As family members are diagnosed with disease, the distance narrows. And as cholesterol or PSA numbers increase, respondents were brought closer to illness. Decreasing these risk numbers fortified the buffer and increased their distance from illness. A weakening of the buffer between health and illness left respondents in a vulnerable position.

Measured vulnerability

Characterising the experience of risk as *measured vulnerability* recognises the lay, and sometimes clinical, tendency to interpret statistical measures of health as pronouncements of current health status and as a projection of future health. Respondents felt physically vulnerable and expressed a vulnerability of identity as well. What is unique about those with elevated cholesterol and PSA levels is that their vulnerability was measured numerically. Respondents were confronted with hard evidence of their compromised health status in the form of a precise numerical level that indicated, to respondents, the potential for the development of serious health consequences. I develop the concept of *measured vulnerability* to characterise how participants experienced risk in their everyday lives.

Vulnerability and uncertainty

When asked how having elevated cholesterol changed the way she thought about her health, Nancy said, 'I guess it makes me feel more vulnerable'. In a similar manner, when Sarah was asked how she would feel if her cholesterol was to fall below 200, she said:

> Safer would be the word . . . I would feel safer knowing that I'm not a walking time bomb, not waiting for something to happen . . . [but] I am no longer in a safe and comfortable thought.

Not only was being at risk something that rendered respondents unable to feel as though they were healthy, there was a sense that illness could befall them at any time, that they were physically vulnerable as a result of their risk numbers.

Marshall held a PhD in engineering and understood how statistics were calculated and could be applied. With that understanding, he said:

> [Being at risk] impacts your sense of your mortality in a way that's very subtle. Even though I don't view these numbers as risky, just the fact that, okay, I've got this thing

that's not in the normal range . . . On the other hand, it's a placeholder for mortality at some point, and there is going to be a time when I get something really bad. And I'm – it's almost like an anticipation, okay, this is the first of what may be a series of 'uh-ohs' down the road, and I think that that – that impact is very subtle, but I think it's real. I think it's a real effect.

Even understanding that having an elevated PSA should not be equated with the presence of cancer, or that it did not mean he was unhealthy, Marshall reported that being at risk led to an anticipation that something was coming that threatened his mortality. And while perhaps very subtle, as Marshall indicated, there can be very real effects as a consequence of being at risk.

Those who are ill often find it difficult to assign meaning to their condition or to predict future outcomes (Weitz 1989, Mishel 1990). Participants who were at risk also experienced significant uncertainty, although the sources of their uncertainty were not always the same as for those who are ill. Being at risk typically produced more questions for respondents, rather than answers.

There are no norms for being at risk. There is no 'risk role', similar to Parsons' Sick Role (Parsons 1951). The unavailability of prescribed social roles that can be adopted by those who are at risk produced uncertainty pertaining to expected behaviours. Respondents were not sure how to react to being at risk emotionally, and were not given clear instructions on how to address their risk status. Respondents were simply unsure how to act.

Beyond an inability to accept being at risk and to understand appropriate social roles, respondents were left with questions about their health that risk numbers left unanswered. Perhaps the most interesting aspect of risk is that it is intended to definitively, numerically, measure the probability of adverse outcomes and provide a tool for management. However, in the lives of those who are at risk, the experience was just the opposite. Probabilities that are based on populations are often used by individuals to determine prospects of future health (Crawford 2004).

Uncertainty was the norm, and this led to fear, anxiety, and uneasiness about the future. As Charles noted, 'That uncertainty is what produces the anxiety, you know, and I don't like that. But what can you do about it?' When I followed up on Charles' comments and asked if additional PSA tests helped to ease the uncertainty he felt, his response was, 'Then that ratchets up the more uncertainty'. Instead of alleviating the uncertainty he experienced, Charles noted that tests only served to give him additional numbers that intensified his uncertainty (see Evans *et al.* 2007, Clark and Talcott 2006).

Uncertainty is a fundamental aspect of the experience of risk. Marshall stated, 'It would not be correct to say I'm living on borrowed time, but I'm living on uncertain time'. The uncertain time on which respondents lived meant that they didn't have a clear sense of what risk meant to their everyday lives or of the implications of being at risk. Instead of leading to certainty and providing direction in managing one's health, risk led to vulnerability and uncertainty. As a numerical measure, it is necessary to understand the meanings of risk numbers and the role of numbers in producing uncertainty.

The meanings of numbers

Deborah Lupton (1995) writes that 'risk discourse depends on its calculability, and quantification and measurement are integral to the discourse and philosophy of risk' (1995: 78). However, risk levels, or thresholds, are not static and are often the product of debate and negotiation within expert communities (Will 2005). Numbers meant different things to those with elevated cholesterol and PSA levels. For those with elevated cholesterol, their numbers indicated thresholds. While the US National Cholesterol Education Program (NCEP 1988) launched the 'Know Your Number' campaign to encourage people to have their cholesterol checked and to know what their numbers were (Greene 2007), it was surprising that many respondents did not have a precise recall of their exact cholesterol numbers.

Some respondents did know their numbers, but most participants were not able to provide an exact total cholesterol number. Instead, they simply stated, 'It was pretty high, I don't remember the numbers' (Peter). Or, 'It was over 200. That was all I cared about' (Susan). Many respondents came up with a cholesterol number, but it was an estimate, or was given as a range.

Respondents with elevated cholesterol thought more in terms of thresholds than precise numbers. Cholesterol thresholds of 'high', or 'borderline-high' represented levels that respondents used as indicators of health. Decreasing cholesterol levels below these thresholds, to 'normal', was interpreted as improving one's health.

It was common for those with elevated cholesterol levels to delay further cholesterol testing until they believed their levels had decreased. Avoiding screenings was a strategy respondents used to minimise the stigma they experienced as a result of their cholesterol levels, with a preference to delay future testing until progress had been made (Frich *et al.* 2007).

Those respondents with elevated PSA levels, on the other hand, were much more likely to have a precise grasp of their PSA numbers. During the interviews, respondents spoke in very specific terms about their numbers. Participants were usually able to recite their numbers, and could do so for past tests as well.

While many respondents with elevated cholesterol indicated that they received their test results in the mail, only one respondent implied that they still had the results somewhere. However, it was striking that most respondents with elevated PSA levels actually produced hard copies of their PSA tests for me to thumb through as we spoke.

In the absence of any national campaign encouraging them to do so, men with elevated PSA levels knew their numbers, and were keeping track. When Tim was asked about his numbers, he consulted his records and said:

It was September of 1998, so just under nine years. 6.1 – that was the first time. Then in December it went down to 5.6 . . . I was on a three-month recall because it was high. In March it spiked to 9.2, was repeated in April, 8.1, had a biopsy. Biopsy was benign. Dropped back and it hovers now, there's a range between – I guess the lowest it's been in the last seven years is 4.4 and the highest it's been since the start of 2000, was 7.3 and it's gone up, it's gone down, it's gone up, it's gone down.

Exchanges similar to this were common during the interviews.

Respondents kept careful track of the trajectory of their PSA levels. Numbers that would bounce around, or that were not consistent, led to uncertainty and anxiety for respondents. Many respondents' concerns centered on the potential need for additional biopsies. Invariably, respondents recounted negative experiences with the prostate biopsy, describing it as a very unpleasant experience.

A spike in one's PSA could be the result of the development of prostate cancer and would be cause for their urologist to recommend a biopsy. Brian noted that his PSA score had spiked and said:

I went up to 5.7. So now I've hit an all time high. I had the atypical ones and now I'm going to go in again for 12 more pieces of tissue. Right? And I'm like, 'I got to have it this time. I've got to have it'.

Additionally, referring to how his PSA tests often lead to other tests, Brian said, 'It's like they cause you to have the biopsy'. Respondents described having a difficult time making sense of their levels, as they were often inconsistent.

Managing uncertainty

Finally, respondents developed strategies for managing the uncertainty that accompanied being at risk. Those facing uncertainty often attempt to assert a measure of control over their treatment (Weitz 1989). As the variability of PSA levels often led to further biopsies, men in the study tracked their PSA scores themselves in an attempt to manage the uncertainty that accompanied their risk status. Monitoring PSA levels and tracking the results was a primary means of managing uncertainty. Respondents' efforts to keep track of their PSA levels represented a method of wresting control from their physicians in order to exert a degree of influence over their care.

Most respondents with elevated cholesterol levels managed their uncertainty by avoiding screening tests, choosing to avoid testing in order to ease the stigma and guilt associated with their risk status that resulted from attributions of personal responsibility for their risk status (Sachs 1996). Many participants said they wanted to wait until they felt as though they had made progress, through lifestyle changes, in their cholesterol levels before they were screened again.

For those with elevated cholesterol levels, being at risk was experienced as vulnerability, which led to uncertainty and anxiety. Rather than focusing on precise numbers, respondents thought in terms of thresholds of risk. Respondents with elevated PSA levels, on the other hand, fixated on precise numbers and tracked the trajectory of their levels in an attempt to manage the uncertainty they felt and to minimise anxiety. It is important to note how these screenings served to intensify the anxiety participants experienced.

The focus on thresholds further demonstrates how respondents visualised a buffer between health and illness. Crossing thresholds, in either direction, became an indication of how close they might be to illness. The more narrow the perceived buffer, the more anxiety and uncertainty respondents experienced.

Discussion and conclusions

Robert Aronowitz (2009) notes how risk has come to be treated like chronic illness, in that being at risk is increasingly viewed as a condition that one will manage indefinitely. He states that the result of this amplified attention to risk will be 'more people who are aware for longer periods of time about possible future ill health and who will be advised to modify their lifestyle and undergo types of surveillance and medical prevention' (2009: 426). As risk comes to resemble chronic illness, it is necessary to account for how people who are at risk experience this new health condition.

While the outcome of chronic illness is often a prolonged period of remission (Frank 1995), being at risk is not necessarily preceded by any compromise in physical functioning. Rather, this new condition may have no symptoms, no lesions, or no identifiable pathology. Instead of a biological entity, being at risk is an epidemiological or probabilistic entity, one that reflects a person's place within a numerical distribution.

Being at risk is an experience in which individuals live with a feeling of measured vulnerability. Characterising the symbolic effects of the risk experience as measured vulnerability recognises the importance of numbers both in the diagnosis of risk and the management of uncertainty, but also specifies the vulnerability that results from the use of numbers to define and manage risk. Numbers were often used by respondents to determine how close they were to becoming ill, or to estimate their personal buffer between health and illness. Putting a number on a person's risk status conveys a sense of certainty, and this was often interpreted as likely or as inevitable.

Measured vulnerability refers to the capacity for scientifically-derived statistical measures that are intended to tame randomness and provide certainty in managing risk to, instead, produce uncertainty and anxiety in those to whom the statistic is applied. Kathleen Woodward (2003) refers to this as 'statistical panic'. She writes that, 'Even when the citation of statistics is meant to provide reassurance, it may more often than not produce its opposite: a sense of foreboding and insecurity' (2003: 226). It is this sense of vulnerability to future ill health that most accurately represents the experiences of those who are at risk. The use of numbers to measure this vulnerability contributes to a reification of the experience of risk. Sulik (2009) refers to this as the development of a technoscientific illness identity. It is important to recognise that health risk is not merely an innocuous application of probabilities. The designation of risk can have a very real impact on the identities of those who have been designated as being at risk.

Measured vulnerability has the conceptual capacity to represent the experiences of those who undergo a shift in their health status as a result of the numerical results of health risk assessments, or screenings. The sense of vulnerability those at risk experience is both quantified and tentative, a combination that results in considerable uncertainty. Measured vulnerability can be a useful concept in symbolising the experience of those who find themselves in the liminal space between health and illness (Navon and Morag 2004, Scott *et al*. 2005, Timmermans and Buchbinder 2010).

This research has significant implications for understanding how people designated as being at risk for health conditions through the presence of genetic factors or other markers experience their health status. Risk factors such as BRCA1/BRCA2 for breast cancer, cancer antigen 125 (CA-125) for ovarian cancer, markers for Huntington's disease, or even having a family history of certain illnesses, do not have associated symptoms or even guarantee the eventual development of disease. It is, however, expected that the potential illness indicated by such risk factors produces an experience that is very similar to the risk experience developed in this research.

Recent controversy surrounding the efficacy of the PSA test has noted the damaging effects of applying risk to people in a way that does not suggest a definitive course of action (Ablin 2010). Dissatisfaction with the specificity of the PSA test has led to the development of the PCA3 urine test that promises to provide more accuracy in the detection of prostate cancer. However, my research suggests that greater statistical certainty does not decrease uncertainty for those who are labelled as being at risk. On the contrary, the result of statistical precision was measured vulnerability.

Respondents with elevated PSA levels did not acknowledge the contested nature of the PSA test in the interviews, which indicated that it was not salient for them. Their experiences should not be considered to be merely a function of poor medical management, or a lack of appropriate education in the physician/patient interaction. Regardless of the intent of medical professionals, respondents felt a sense of measured vulnerability as a result of their risk status.

While physicians may recognise the limited value of the PSA (or cholesterol) test, their patients use these test results differently, using the numbers as placeholders for health. However, this is an area that should be studied further. My research does not address the role of physicians in making a designation of risk for those with elevated cholesterol and PSA levels. A better appreciation of this interaction would contribute to a more detailed understanding of the experiences of those who are at risk.

It may be the case that as individuals are better able to quantify the buffer between health and illness they will experience a more intense feeling of vulnerability. This inverse relationship between statistical precision and measured vulnerability will be an important consideration in evaluating risk screening tests that continue to emerge. As screening becomes the primary method of assessing health status by health professionals, lay persons will increasingly rely upon the results of these screening tests to assess their personal buffers to illness. Exploring the relationship between the application of risk and the experience of risk promises to add greater understanding to how individuals process information that is derived from populations.

Acknowledgements

I would like to thank Peter Conrad, Stefan Timmermans, and Cheryl Stults for comments and insights in the development of this essay. I would also like to thank the Editors and reviewers for providing direction and very useful feedback.

References

Ablin, R.J. (2010) The great prostate mistake, *New York Times*, 9 March, OpEd.

Armstrong, D. (1995) The rise of surveillance medicine, *Sociology of Health and Illness*, 17, 3, 393–404.

Aronowitz, R. (1998) *Making Sense of Illness: Science, Society, and Disease*. Cambridge: Cambridge University Press.

Aronowitz, R. (2009) The convergence experience of risk and disease, *The Milbank Quarterly*, 87, 2, 417–42.

Arnst, C. (1999) The risk of disease will be treated as a disease, *Business Week* (3644).

Brown, J., Chapman, S. and Lupton, D. (1996) Infinitesimal risk as public health crisis: news media coverage of a doctor-patient HIV contact tracing investigation, *Social Science and Medicine*, 43, 12, 1685–95.

Bury, M. (1982) Chronic illness as biograhical disruption, *Sociology of Health and Illness*, 4, 2, 167–82.

Bury, M. (1991) The sociology of chronic illness: a review of research and prospects, *Sociology of Health and Illness*, 13, 4, 451–68.

Catalona, W.J. (1992) Single and serial measurement of serum prostate-specific antigen as a screening test for early prostate cancer, *Journal of Urology*, 147, 450A.

Charmaz, K. (1983) Loss of self: a fundamental form of suffering in the chronically ill, *Sociology of Health and Illness*, 5, 2, 168–95.

Charmaz, K. (1987) Struggling for a self: identity levels of the chronically ill. In Roth, J.A. and Conrad, P. (eds) *Research in the Sociology of Health Care*. Greenwich, CT: JAI Press.

Clark, J.A. and Talcott, J.A. (2006) Confidence and uncertainty long after initial treatment for early prostate cancer: survivors' views of cancer control and the treatment decisions they made, *Journal of Clinical Oncology*, 24, 27, 4457–63.

Clarke, E., Mamo, L., Fishman, J.R., *et al.* (2003) Biomedicalization: technoscientific transformations of health, illness, and U.S. biomedicine, *American Sociological Review*, 68, April, 161–94.

Conrad, P. (1985) The meaning of medications: another look at compliance, *Social Science and Medicine*, 20, 1, 29–37.

Conrad, P. (2007) *The Medicalization of Society*. Baltimore, Md.: Johns Hopkins University Press.

Crawford, R. (2004) Risk ritual and the management of control and anxiety in medical culture, *Health*, 8, 4, 505–28.

Eastham, J., Riedel, E., Scardino, P.T., *et al.* (2003) Variation of serum prostate-specific antigen levels: an evaluation of year-to-year fluctuation, *JAMA*, 289, 20, 2695–700.

Evans, R., Edwards, A.G., Elwyn, G., *et al.* (2007) 'It's a Maybe Test': men's experience of prostate specific antigen testing in primary care, *British Journal of General Practice*, 57, 303–10.

Foucault, M. (1988) Technologies of the self. In Martin, L.H., Gutman, H. and Hutton, P.H. (eds) *Technologies of the Self.* Amhert: University of Massachusetts Press.

Foucault, M. (1991) Governmentality. In Burchell, G., Gardon, C. and Miller, P. (eds) *The Foucault Effect: Studies in Governmentality*. Chicago: University of Chicago Press.

Fowler, F.J. (2006) The impact of a suspicious prostate biopsy on patients' psychological, socio-behavioral, and medical care outcomes, *Journal of General Internal Medicine*, 21, 7, 715–21.

Frank, A. (1995) *The Wounded Storyteller: Body, Illness, and Ethics*. Chicago: University of Chicago Press.

Frich, J. (2007) Experiences of guilt and shame in patients with familial hypercholesterolemia: a qualitative interview study, *Patient Education and Counseling*, 69, 1–3, 108–13.

Garrety, K. (1998) Science, policy, and controversy in the cholesterol arena, *Symbolic Interaction*, 21, 4, 401–24.

Greaves, D. (2000) The creation of partial patients, *Cambridge Quarterly of Healthcare Ethics*, 9, 23–37.

Greene, J. (2007) *Prescribing by Numbers*. Baltimore: Johns Hopkins University Press.

Goffman, E. (1963) *Stigma: Notes on the Management of a Spoiled Identity*. Englewood Cliffs, NJ: Prentice-Hall.

Goffman, E. (1967) *Interaction Ritual*. New York: Pantheon.

Kabat, G.C. (2008) *Hyping Health Risks: Environmental Hazards in Daily Life and the Science of Epidemiology*. New York: Columbia University Press.

Keeley, B., Wright, L. and Condit, C.M. (2009) Functions of health and fatalism: fatalistic talk as face saving, uncertainty management, stress relief and sense making, *Sociology of Health and Illness*, 31, 5, 734–47.

Lidskog, R. (1996) In science we trust? On the relation between scientific knowledge, risk consciousness and public trust, *Acta Sociologica*, 39, 1, 31–56.

Lupton, D. (1995) *The Imperative of Health: Public Health and the Regulated Body*. London: Sage.

Lupton, D. (1999) *Risk*. London: Routledge.

Meyers, G. (2003) Risk and face: a review of the six studies, *Health, Risk and Society*, 5, 2, 215–20.

Mishel, M.H. (1990) Reconceptualization of the uncertainty in illness theory, *IMAGE: Journal of Nursing Scholarship*, 22, 4, 256–62.

National Center for Health Statistics. (2009) *Health, 2008, United States with Chartbook*. Hyattsville: Md.

National Cholesterol Education Panel. (1988) Report of the national cholesterol education program expert panel on detection, evaluation, and treatment of high blood cholesterol in adults, *Archives of Internal Medicine*, 148, 36–69.

National Cholesterol Education Panel. (2001) *Third Report of the National Cholesterol Education Program (NCEP) Expert Panel on Detection, Evaluation, and Treatment of High Blood Cholesterol in Adults (Adult Treatment Panel III) – Executive Summary*, National Heart, Lung, and Blood Institute.

Navon, L. and Morag, A. (2004) Liminality as biographical disruption: unclassifiability following hormonal therapy for advanced prostate cancer, *Social Science and Medicine*, 58, 11, 2337–47.

Nelkin, D. (1989) Communicating technological risk: the social construction of risk perception, *Annual Review of Public Health*, 10, 95–113.

Nerlich, B. and Koteyko, N. (2008) Balancing food risks and food benefits: the coverage of probiotics in the UK national press, *Sociological Research Online*, 13, 3, 21.

Nettleton, S., Burrows, R. and Watt, I. (2005) The mundane realities of the everyday lay use of the internet for health, and their consequences for media convergence, *Sociology of Health and Illness*, 27, 7, 972–92.

Paterson, B. (2001) The shifting perspectives model of chronic illness, *Journal of Nursing Scholarship*, 33, 1, 21–6.

Pound, P. (2005) Resisting medicines: a synthesis of qualitative studies of medicine taking, *Social Science and Medicine*, 61, 1, 133–55.

Rosenberg, C. (2009) Managed fear, *The Lancet*, 373, 802–03.

Sachs, L. (1996) Causality, responsibility and blame – core issues in the cultural construction and subtext of prevention, *Sociology of Health and Illness*, 18, 5, 632–52.

Schneider, J.W. and Conrad, P. (1983) *Having Epilepsy: the Experience and Control of Illness*. Philadelphia, PA: Temple University Press.

Scott, S., Prior, L., Wood, F. and Gray, J. (2005) Repositioning the patient: the implications of being 'at-risk', *Social Science and Medicine*, 60, 8, 1869–79.

Siegrist, M., Keller, C., Kastenholz, H., *et al.* (2007) Laypeople's and experts' perception of nanotechnology hazards, *Risk Analysis*, 27, 1, 59–69.

Sulik, G. (2009) Managing biomedical uncertainty: the techonoscientific illness identity, *Sociology of Health and Illness*, 31, 7, 1059–76.

Timmermans, S. and Buchbinder, M. (2010) Patients-in-waiting: living between sickness and health in the genomics era, *Journal of Health and Social Behavior*, 51, 4, 408–23.

Weiss, M. (1997) Signifying the pandemics: metaphors of AIDS, cancer, and heart disease, *Medical Anthropology Quarterly*, 11, 4, 456–76.

Weitz, R. (1989) Uncertainty and the lives of persons with AIDS, *Journal of health & social behavior*, 30, 3, 270–81.

Will, C. (2005) Arguing about the evidence: readers, writers and inscription devices in coronary heart disease assessment, *Sociology of Health and Illness*, 27, 6, 780–801.

Williams, S. (2000) Chronic Illness as biographical disruption or biological disruption as chronic illness? Reflection on a core concept, *Sociology of Health and Illness*, 22, 5, 40–67.

Woodward, K. (1999) Statistical panic, *Differences: a Journal of Feminist Cultural Studies*, 11, 2, 178–203.

Woodward, K. (2003) The Statistical body. In Coupland, J. and Gwyn, R. (eds) *Discourse, the Body, and Identity*. London: Palgrave Macmillan.

4

Expanded newborn screening: articulating the ontology of diseases with bridging work in the clinic
Stefan Timmermans and Mara Buchbinder

Introduction

Screening large populations for diseases has a powerful humanitarian rationale that appeals to medical professionals, public health authorities and health policymakers (Rose 1992). Screening follows the logic of secondary prevention: a population is screened to detect disease early and to initiate treatment before symptoms emerge. However, not all population screening is justifiable under all circumstances. In the 1960s the World Health Organization formulated the gold standard for initiating a population-screening programme. Realising the opportunity costs of investing in expensive screening programmes, Wilson and Jungner argued that one should invest in screening only if the screened condition constitutes 'an important health problem' with accessible treatment; a discriminating screening test that is acceptable to the general population is available; an 'adequate' understanding of the condition's natural history exists, and screening offers a favourable cost-benefit ratio (Wilson and Jungner, 1968: 26–7).

In this article, we unpack Wilson and Jungner's requirement that knowledge about the natural history of a disease must be adequate for screening to proceed. We argue that any prior understanding of disease is inevitably found to be insufficient once population screening is instituted. As clinicians and public health researchers have learned from population screening for phenylketonuria (Paul 1997), sickle cell anemia (Wailoo and Pemberton 2006) and other conditions, once screening is implemented, uncertainty emerges because the diseases do not behave as expected based on previous scientific knowledge. Screening produces anomalous findings in light of what clinicians thought they knew about the conditions. These unexpected findings encompass all of the dimensions Wilson and Jungner cover: disease incidence, severity, the distinction between pathological and benign variations and response to treatment. The findings provoke the fundamental question: what is the nature of the condition we are screening for? Yet, as we will show, clinicians help bridge the ontological gap between pre-screening and post-screening knowledge.

The nature of various metabolic diseases has recently been questioned in the USA with the expansion of newborn screening. In 2006 the American College of Medical Genetics (ACMG) expanded newborn screening by advocating the adoption of new technologies that allow simultaneous screening for multiple conditions (Watson et al. 2006). The ACMG

The Sociology of Medical Screening, First Edition. Edited by Natalie Armstrong and Helen Eborall.
Chapters © 2012 The Authors. Book Compilation © 2012 Foundation for the Sociology of Health & Illness / Blackwell Publishing Ltd. Published 2012 by Blackwell Publishing Ltd.

recommended screening for a panel of 29 core conditions and 25 secondary conditions that would be identified incidentally when screening for the core set. In only a few years, all 50 states implemented the new technologies and most began screening for the recommended panel. Now, a blood sample of virtually all the 4.25 million infants born in the USA each year is sent to a state-contracted laboratory, which, in turn, will notify paediatricians, geneticists and families when they find positive results.

When anxious mothers and fathers hold seemingly normal infants in their arms after being told that their child screened positive for a rare metabolic condition, determining the clinical implications of a positive screen carries an existential urgency. Rather than playing a secondary role in the era of evidence-based medicine (Timmermans and Berg 2003a), the clinic re-emerges as a site of knowledge production (Latimer *et al.* 2006, Rabeharisoa and Bourret 2009). For rare genetic diseases, randomised clinical trial data are non-existent and even clinical experience is in short supply. Clinicians and parents face a profound practical and moral problem of what to do about this baby whose biochemical levels lie outside a preset normal range.

Drawing upon ethnographic research conducted in a California regional clinical centre for metabolic-genetic disorders, we examine how the clinic staff collectively performs what we call bridging work to gradually revise their understanding of the clinical nature of conditions unsettled by population-based newborn screening. Generally, bridging work refers to the many activities required to reconcile the promise of technologies with the realities of their implementation. The introduction of new technologies affects a workplace at multiple levels, including the incorporation of technology into available health services, the divisions of labour between medical subspecialties and, importantly, the lives of beneficiaries and others affected directed and indirectly by the technology. Here, we highlight work done in the clinic to align the epistemic or knowledge properties of diseases: work involving an ontological transformation of diseases following the introduction of technologies.

In line with the social studies of science literature (Kuhn 1962), we refer to unexpected findings related to the knowledge properties of screened conditions as anomalies because these findings are unusual in light of the scientific knowledge base prior to the implementation of new technologies. These anomalies require identification and remedial work to incorporate the technology into work practices. In the case of screening, newly adopted screening technologies are supposed to detect well-known diseases but instead produce biomedical information that no longer fits the knowledge base. Clinicians reconcile the gap between what was known about a disease prior to screening and the outcomes of population screening. The result is an ontological transformation of disease categories. We centre our discussion on the reconfiguration of medium chain acyl-CoA dehydrogenase deficiency (MCADD), a disorder that served as a catalyst for expanded newborn screening.

We are also interested in how the knowledge generated about diseases affects the rationale for population-based screening. The disease characteristics that help justify population screening are also cast into doubt with the implementation of screening. However, even when the cost-benefit analysis of population screening shifts, it is difficult to turn back the screening momentum precisely because the work in the clinic buffers ontological incompatibilities.

The clinic as centre of knowledge production

Diseases change. They are not stable objects but are transformed based on the practices they become part of (Mol 2002). They change not simply in the patient groups they affect but also ontologically and epistemologically: what we understand as a specific disease and how we know about a disease. Historians have examined how signs and symptoms are grouped differently over time, rendering dissimilar physical and mental processes visible, shifting causal processes, implicating novel patient groups and relating differently to professional practices and healthcare systems (Aronowitz 2008, Rosenberg 2007). Key examples include homosexuality in psychiatry (Kirk and Kutchins 1992), the radical changed understanding of HIV-AIDS over a 10-year period (Epstein 1996) and the transformation of cystic fibrosis and heart disease over the past century (Greene 2007, Kerr 2005). In fact, the notion that people suffer from a specific disease – rather than an imbalance between an individual and the environment – is itself a historical achievement of medical thinking that dates back to the late 18th century (Rosenberg 2007).

Ontological and epistemological changes in diseases may occur gradually or be provoked by technological innovations. Technological catalysts include pharmaceuticals in search of a disease target (Greene 2007, Lakoff 2005), the creation of new classification systems or guidelines for disease detection (Bowker and Star 1999), the development of diagnostic tools (Kerr 2005) or, as we argue here, the introduction of population-based screening programmes. Such technological change agents are insufficient to consolidate new realities for diseases. Social scientists have noted that new disease categories require massive social movements to build the infrastructure needed to operationalise disease categories as feasible clinical entities and link potential patients to diagnostic and treatment modalities (for example, Armstrong 1979). Throughout this process the understanding of what the disease is – its natural history, severity, patient groups, treatment response – and the possibilities for action are also transformed.

Even in genetics, where most knowledge about disease susceptibility depends on specific laboratory tests, the ontological properties of diseases are often established in the clinic. Latimer *et al.* (2006) observed how genetic dysmorphologists actively generate, debate and evaluate categories of genetic classification rather than applying externally produced molecular or cytogenetic laboratory knowledge. Observations of dysmorphology and other perceptual clues may qualify genetic findings. Similarly, in oncology and psychiatric genetic clinics, the implementation of molecular medicine 'far from reifying and simplifying pathological situations, expand[s] and recompose[s] them in different ways' (Rabeharisoa and Bourret 2009: 699). This continued role for the clinic in the production of genetic knowledge is not simply a temporary placeholder until technologies provide more definitive tests. Instead, the promise of each new test to resolve ambiguity remains deferred until clinicians determine how and when to use genetic knowledge (Hedgecoe 2004). Rethinking ontological properties may lead to fragmentation or even devaluing the condition's disease status (Mol 2002). The clinic thus remains a site of knowledge production where anomalous findings are worked out.

Setting and methodology

In California, the setting of our research, expanded newborn screening was implemented in 2005. Newborn screening begins within 48 hours after birth, when a blood spot is collected through a prick to the newborn's heel. Tandem mass spectrometry is used to analyse the sample to determine the concentration of specific chemical compounds in the blood. If the value lies outside a predetermined normal range, metabolic disease is a possibility and the child's paediatrician will order a follow-up test. If the results still suggest disease, the family will be referred to a regional clinical centre for further follow-up testing and, if indicated, treatment.

Our analysis is based on close observations of clinical interactions between parents and the genetics team, which consisted of four medical geneticists, three genetic counsellors, a nurse practitioner clinical coordinator, a dietitian and a social worker. We followed parents during clinic visits over a three year period (October 2007 to July 2010). In the metabolic-genetics clinic we audio-recorded consultations between parents and genetics staff with a research team member present to observe the interaction and take ethnographic field notes. In addition, we attended weekly staff meetings and consulted patient records. The project received Institutional Review Board approval.

All English-speaking and Spanish-speaking families of clinic patients who received a positive newborn screen between 2007 and 2009 were approached for participation in the study during routine clinic visits. Five families refused to participate because they declined to be audio-recorded and one family was ineligible because they spoke neither Spanish nor English. The families of 75 patients participated in the study. We recorded a total of 193 patient visits, with one to twelve visits recorded per patient. In 16 of the families Spanish was the primary language.

We analysed our data in a modified grounded theory and analytical induction tradition (Timmermans and Tavory 2007), meaning that we systematically coded the empirical material in dialogue with a close reading of salient themes in the medical sociology and genetics literature. Our data analysis approach demands a concerted effort to find negative cases. In addition to the literature on genetics, we also draw from the sociology of work and from science and technology studies. We began the analysis early in the project and verified the emerging analytical coding scheme with later data to make sure that our analysis captured the full spectrum of empirical manifestations.

Findings

Anomalies due to population screening

Prior to newborn screening, clinicians in our study and across the world gathered knowledge about rare metabolic conditions predominantly from symptomatic patients. Often, these patients developed serious complications before a diagnosis was even possible. Diagnostic criteria, biochemical tests, treatment protocols and incidence figures – if available at all – were based on these symptomatic patients. Population screening has demonstrated that such a symptomatic population constituted a biased knowledge base due to under-diagnosis or misdiagnosis prior to screening, declining penetrance, or because the unknown variants are sufficiently rare to remain undiscovered. Consequently, newborn screening expanded the patient base of screening targets by identifying patients prospectively, while they were still asymptomatic. The question facing clinicians was whether the patients identified through newborn screening were similar enough to the symptomatic patients with whom they were familiar to need to be managed with similar protocols. When the incidence figures detected via screening programmes reached much higher levels than expected based on symptomatic patient groups and when the biological indicators among the positive screening patients differed from those of symptomatic patients, clinicians suspected that not all of the patients identified were truly at risk for complications: the conditions were likely to be more hetero-geneous than had been thought prior to screening. Such anomalous findings called into question every step of the disease process from diagnosis to treatment.

Geneticists aimed to reduce the impact of these unexpected findings with bridging work. Such work involved recognising anomalous findings in the context of the prevailing under-standings of screening targets; collectively negotiating the parameters of the anomaly;

developing new knowledge about conditions, and formulating operating procedures to manage the changed disease ontology. Bridging work in the clinic entailed creating and implementing knowledge properties in specific patients' care. We examine this multifaceted work with respect to MCADD diagnosis, disease incidence and severity, therapeutics and outcomes.

The processes of knowledge production are ongoing and the face of MCADD is likely to change again by the time this chapter is published. Rather than pinning down precisely what MCADD is, we draw attention to the ongoing clinical bridging work that transformed knowledge properties.

MCADD

MCADD, first identified in 1982, has been repeatedly presented as the prototype disease for the expansion of newborn screening. With little symptom development, the natural history of this condition was not well understood but the prospect of death as an initial manifestation and an uncomplicated treatment made a compelling case for screening. Despite it being the model for expanded newborn screening, even this most common of the fatty oxidation disorders was transformed with the advent of screening.

MCADD is caused by mutations in the ACADM gene that can cause shortages of medium-chain acyl-coenzyme A dehydrogenase, an enzyme required to metabolise medium-chain fatty acids. This enzymatic deficiency can result in the improper metabolisation of medium-chain fatty acids and their accumulation in the blood, which in turn may cause lethargy, hypoglycemia and liver and brain damage. The primary threat for such metabolic crises is a prolonged period of fasting, which, if left untreated, may result in death. MCADD thus constitutes a predisposition to disease requiring a second trigger of metabolic stress to produce symptoms.

Prior to newborn screening, MCADD patients usually came to medical attention with an episode of severe lethargy or even coma due to hypoglycemia. Mortality rates during such episodes hovered around 25 per cent and another 20–40 per cent of survivors suffered significant morbidity, including irreversible neurological impairments or developmental delays (Iafolla et al. 1994). According to the prevailing wisdom prior to newborn screening, MCADD occurred due to a founder effect most common among non-Hispanic white populations of north-west European descent.

The treatment for MCADD was a low-fat diet and, above all, to avoid fasting and be particularly vigilant when the infant becomes ill and stops eating. Occasionally, clinicians prescribed additional dietary measures such as carnitine supplements or drinking a corn-starch solution – a slow-metabolising carbohydrate – before bedtime or in the middle of the night. If the child vomited repeatedly and could not keep food down, geneticists recommended that parents take the child to an emergency department to receive intravenous glucose. Most symptoms occurred before the age of six, a period of rapid development, but adult onset remained a possibility.

Diagnosis: In clinical consultations, we observed knowledge in the making in tandem with a shifting biomedical literature: what had been viewed as a more or less homogeneous disease, newborn screening unsettled. The first contested issue was what qualified as an MCADD diagnosis. Tests working at different levels of analysis produced different possibilities for diagnosis and these differences needed to be reconciled. In the recent past, patients identified with MCADD exhibited clinical signs and symptoms that were then confirmed by biochemical testing. The combination of clinical symptoms and biochemical findings was sufficient to establish the diagnosis, but physicians could confirm the diagnosis with genetic mutation analysis. Before the introduction of population screening, about

80 per cent of patients were homozygous and about 18 per cent heterozygous for the c.985A > G mutation (Gregersen *et al.* 1993). Since symptoms were already present and the child was obviously affected by the condition, genetic testing did not offer therapeutic value. MCADD was thus a disease in which physical symptoms signalled a biochemical abnormality that corresponded to a common genetic profile. A 2001 study identified a second mutation, c.199T > C, which the authors described as a 'mild folding mutation that exhibits decreased levels of enzyme activity only under stringent condition' (Andresen *et al.* 2001: 1408).

The consistency between symptoms, biochemistry and genetics was undone by population screening. With screening, the entry point for an MCADD diagnosis is a biochemical value, rather than clinical evidence of a metabolic disorder. In our study, all newborn screening patients suspected of having MCADD were asymptomatic. The main indication that an infant might have MCADD was an elevated C8-acylcarnitine level.[1] The anomaly requiring bridging work in the clinic was whether all abnormal biochemical levels constituted pathology in the absence of symptoms or whether some screening results reflected incidental finding without clinical implications. Here, genetic testing gained importance because the prevailing knowledge suggested that the c.199T > C mutation had milder pathogenic effects than the c.985A > G mutation. Screening thus separated symptoms from biochemical indicators and turned genetic data into the arbiter.

We observed the construction of a bridge, the increased reliance on genetic testing to determine the severity of MCADD, when a geneticist early on in our research urged a family to consent to DNA analysis. At the time the newborn screening programme did not cover the cost of mutation analysis for MCADD. The geneticist's plea was complicated by his acknowledgment that the results would not impact on treatment. Nevertheless, the family consented and the results showed that their daughter was heterozygous for the c.985A > G and the c.199T > C mutation. The geneticist presented this as 'reassuring news' because 'nobody who's had this [c.199T > C] mutation found on newborn screening has yet turned up to have an acute episode due to MCADD'. From then on he urged his colleagues to conduct DNA analysis routinely and not to rely on biochemical levels. Genetic testing offered an added therapeutic value because it allowed for a more precise prognosis. This strategy seemed to pay off when the c.199T > C mutation was identified in a large number of patients identified with elevated C8 levels. Because of these experiences, the geneticists in our study successfully advocated for state reimbursement of mutation analysis for the common MCADD mutations. Therefore, bridging work became integrated not only into the clinic's workflow but also into state policy.

However, genetic testing for MCADD was helpful in making a diagnosis only when the results confirmed the two most common mutations. Initial DNA analysis specifically targeted these mutations, but following population screening, DNA testing also identified previously unknown variants. About a year into our study a second geneticist ordered a test for the two common MCADD mutations for a patient that had screened positive at birth. The results came back negative. The geneticist was prepared to dismiss the patient as a likely carrier when, at the insistence of the nurse coordinator, he screened the full gene. He found that the patient was homozygous for a mutation that was at that point unknown. Unknown genetic information did not clarify the clinical significance of the biochemical elevations. In fact, it was unclear whether such mutations were pathogenic for MCADD. In one family where the baby had one known and one unknown mutation, the geneticist ordered mutation analysis for both parents to see whether the person who passed on the unknown mutation manifested metabolic disease. If the parent with the mutation had high C8 levels, the geneticist would know that the mutation is causative for MCADD. The father had a single copy of the unknown mutation but no elevated levels. This information had limited value because it failed to confirm that symptoms could occur with the unknown mutation. The geneticist explained the current status of MCADD diagnosis to the parents as follows:

> Newborn screening has opened up a whole new era of research on the molecular basis of this condition because now the original test just measures the fats, right. So now we're finding that we cannot sometimes just diagnose the condition just based on that. So we have to go to the DNA test, which is what we did in your case. And when we do that, we find all sorts of new mutations that have never been seen before because the cases are probably milder and so we never saw them before.

Thus, MCADD transformed from a disease with consistency between symptoms, metabolic levels and genetic mutations into a condition for which these levels no longer correlated and clinical consequences had been cast into doubt. Genetic testing, long believed to be the definitive indicator of clinical significance, could now aggravate uncertainty when the mutations had unknown clinical significance. The geneticists' bridging work to overcome these ontological uncertainties relied upon the general modus operandi of professionals faced with a situation lacking a scientifically agreed upon course of action. The geneticist here acts as Schutzian ideal type of a 'well-informed citizen' rather than expert. This person exhibits a 'natural attitude' or 'thinking as usual' that consists of a set of stock practical typifications and recipes for action (Schutz 1967). When confronted with anomalous newborn screening results geneticists responded with more precise follow-up genetic testing. Additional bridging work was required when geneticists accustomed to finding clarity from molecular genetics ran into unfamiliar territory. 'DNA sequencing', a geneticist explained to a family, 'can either tell us a lot of information or not give us conclusive information'.

Severity and incidence: An increased reliance on genetic testing to interpret the meaning of biochemical elevations in asymptomatic patients required geneticists to revise their knowledge of the severity and incidence of MCADD. At a 2010 staff meeting, a geneticist in our study mentioned an article that had taken stock of five years of gene sequencing following newborn screening at the Mayo Clinic. The authors noted that newborn screening revealed several 'ACADM variants of unknown significance for which it is not clear whether the DNA variants are rare polymorphisms or pathogenic mutations' (Smith et al. 2010: 241). MCADD broke down into 'carrier-like', 'intermediate' and 'severe' variants (Smith et al. 2010: 245). Carrier-like meant that an individual inherited a genetic trait but did not exhibit symptoms associated with the mutation. The intermediate level implied a degree of functional deficiency that required treatment and clinical follow up although the clinical risk remained unclear, while the severe form suggested a higher clinical risk although patients with 'severe' variants may remain asymptomatic (Smith et al. 2010: 245, 248). To distinguish between these three types, the authors correlated 75 genetic mutations – many of which had not been previously documented – with a broad array of biochemical findings including the concentration of C8 in blood plasma, the C8:C2 and C8:C10 ratio and the excretion of hexanoylglycine (HG) in urine.[2] The geneticists in our study treated this study as a new bridge to deal with the problem of genotypic variants with unknown clinical significance. They referred to it as an algorithm for dealing with unknown mutations and as evidence for an intermediate level of MCADD. In this case, bridging work involved bringing the scientific literature to bear on the experience of clinical uncertainty, resulting in an expanded set of biochemical criteria for defining MCADD.

What qualified as common MCADD also needed revision. Prior to newborn screening, researchers estimated that 80–90 per cent of MCADD patients had the c.985A > G mutation of the ACADM gene but following the implementation of screening programmes in Germany, Australia and the USA the incidence has been downgraded to about 50 per cent (Maier *et al.* 2005, Waddell *et al.* 2006). The same newborn screening experiences also suggested that while the c.985A > G mutation is more common among north Europeans, other populations may have different MCADD mutations and the worldwide incidence of the condition is approximately twice as high as previously thought (Maier *et al.* 2005). One couple in our study hoped that their child might not have MCADD because the father was eastern European and the mother Mexican, and they had read on the internet that 'this is mostly a northern European trait'. However, the geneticist indicated that such information was quickly becoming outdated. Indeed, he cited the Mayo study to interpret the patient's mutation: 'the c.443G > A variant is frequent among individuals with Latin American ancestry' (Smith *et al.* 2010: 247).

Due to newborn screening, MCADD proliferates. There are not only more asymptomatic cases but more MCADD variants exist alongside each other. Inevitably, such heterogeneity provokes important questions about which variants constitute real cases of disease or whether MCADD is too diverse to be considered a single disease. Here, proliferation does not lead to ontological disintegration because the geneticists work to maintain a common identity across the MCADD variants. Clinicians reclassify and rank the patients and corresponding MCADD variants along a continuum of severity based upon their genetic and metabolic profile.

Treatment: The ontological transformation and expansion of the MCADD category did not affect treatment protocols. Geneticists erred on the side of caution by sticking to the pre-screening treatment protocol despite post-screening MCADD differentiation. The standardised treatment protocol further helped to maintain a singular identity for MCADD and indirectly addressed some of the confusion about the changing nature of MCADD post-screening. This uniform treatment regimen worked for MCADD because the treatment was non-invasive; it rested upon vigilance during periods of reduced food intake, regular feedings with a low-fat diet and, occasionally, dietary supplements. The treatment depended upon education: the geneticist instructed the parents to go to the closest emergency department if the child became ill and could not eat and issued an emergency letter for parents to share with hospital staff. The genetic staff strategically deployed a uniform treatment protocol in spite of MCADD variation to authoritatively address the parental distress caused by newborn screening results (Buchbinder and Timmermans 2011, Timmermans and Buchbinder 2010). This move conveyed the view that, while there might be uncertainty about the clinical variation of MCADD, they knew how to treat all cases effectively.

The basic treatment regimen did not vary regardless of the severity suggested by genetic mutations and biochemical levels. When the test results for one patient showed a heterozygous mutation, the geneticist warned that the parents should not get 'cocky' over these results because their child was not disease free: 'Obviously, if she pukes her guts out one day, you really want to take more precautions than you would take for the child who didn't have this'. Regardless of the severity of the condition, the geneticist reminded the parents not to let the baby fast for more than four to eight hours and to be especially vigilant if the infant was ill and, more particularly, vomiting. A geneticist summarised the knowledge about treatment as:

> it turns out that the only thing that we know for sure prevents the adverse consequences of this is not letting the kids fast for a long time. All the other [treatments] appear to be window dressing.

With this treatment regimen in place, geneticists adapted less critical recommendations to a changing consensus in their field. For example, the maximum number of hours that MCADD patients were advised to go without food evolved over the course of our study. Initially, the geneticists told parents of MCADD patients to feed their newborn every two to three hours and to keep up this regime until the sixth month. Informed by an international listserve, the geneticists changed their recommendation to adding 1 extra hour for each month of the infant's age. Thus, a four-month old could sleep for four hours uninterrupted and a six-month old for six hours. The limit of uninterrupted sleep was set at eight hours. We observed other preventative measures relax over the course of our study, again, regardless of the severity of the MCADD. Some of the patients diagnosed with MCADD soon after newborn screening was implemented had been instructed to drink a cornstarch solution before bedtime to provide extra energy during the night. Over time, the geneticists no longer thought this was necessary for most of the MCADD patients.

The geneticists used the ambiguity in treatment regimens strategically: they erred on the side of caution but also adjusted less critical preventive measures in response to parents' concerns. With some parents, the geneticist negotiated the number of hours the child could sleep, responding to parents' reluctance to wake a sleeping baby. A geneticist told the parents of a four-month-old boy whom the parents preferred to let sleep: 'We just have to reach a compromise. I'm happy to reach a medium of five [hours of sleep] but not more than that'. The compromise showed responsiveness to parental desires and conveyed the message that MCADD should not be underestimated. The number of hours of sleep was a negotiable preventive treatment: geneticists realised that the 1 hour per month was chosen largely for its heuristic and mnemonic value. Some parents preferred to hold to stricter preventive measures to strengthen their child's safety net. Thus, when a geneticist heard that the parents of a 5-year-old boy were still giving him cornstarch at night, he pointed out that the dose the boy was receiving was quite low:

> That's probably under-dosed. Let me tell you: no one agrees whether it's a useful treatment or not. So, there's several ways to deal with this. One way is to just stop it and measure it and there is another way, which is just to leave him at the same dose and then at some point in 2 years from now, it'll be so under-dosed that then you'll be able to just stop it.

The physician realised that asking a family to eliminate a preventive treatment that they had been using for years could be a difficult proposition. Instead, he opted to gradually phase out the treatment to the point where its effects would no longer be therapeutic, giving the parents time to adjust and to accept that their child was likely to be fine.

Generally, the uniform treatment regimen regardless of MCADD variation indirectly addressed some of the anomalies in the knowledge base produced by newborn screening. The geneticists' actions conveyed the view that, despite uncertainties about whether every mutation and biochemical abnormality is pathological, the treatment is straightforward and effective. Bridging work in the treatment area thus involved maintaining pre-screening knowledge in spite of changed MCADD ontology.

Outcomes: In an earlier version of this chapter we wrote that for all the ontological revisions of the nature of MCADD, newborn screening had succeeded in preventing the onset of serious disease. We based our assessment on a review by Australian geneticist Wilcken who reviewed the literature on MCADD health outcomes after newborn screening and concluded 'there is very little risk of death after diagnosis [and] the risk of intellectual deficit or other morbidities in survivors is small' (Wilcken 2010: 501, 503). The geneticists in our study echoed this message to reassure anxious parents. One patient required a hospitalisation but she also stabilised quickly after the emergency room staff administered glucose intravenously, which provided further proof to the genetic staff that MCADD is effectively treatable. The proliferation of carrier-like and intermediate MCADD increasingly seemed to suggest that most of the MCADD cases revealed by expanded newborn screening lay at the milder end of the spectrum.

In September 2010, however, the genetics staff became aware of a study showing that some infants with MCADD have died even after newborn screening diagnosis and close medical surveillance (Yusopov *et al.* 2010). The nurse coordinator, who forwarded us the article, described it as 'scary stuff'. She wanted to call the parents of all of her MCADD patients to tell them to be very cautious, especially when the child vomited. This article once again modified the MCADD knowledge base and encouraged the genetics staff to impress on families the even greater urgency to seek medical care at the first signs of illness. This article may prompt bridging work for a different set of anomalies. Rather than employing uncertainties to reassure, the staff may deploy the same uncertainties to alert families to unpredictable dangers. Bridging work, then, consists of continuously working out unexpected results in the clinic, as they emerge in real time.

Discussion and conclusion

MCADD, the poster child for the expansion of newborn screening, became ontologically undone after population screening. From a singular disease it morphed into a condition with carrier-like, intermediate and severe variants. Population screening undermined the tight links between molecular, metabolic and phenotypic disease indicators, created new classifications and utilities for various metabolic indicators and identified new kinds of patients with different risk factors. And, generally, the incidence of the condition was much higher than anticipated and included patients of more diverse ethnicities. For clinicians who had learned that MCADD is a potentially fatal disease that is found in non-Hispanic whites, the repeated identification of asymptomatic MCADD patients of diverse ethnicities required a revision of the nature of MCADD. The ontological reshuffle did not reach a crisis situation for the screening programme because of the bridging work in the clinic.

Wilson and Jungner proposed that the knowledge of a disease should be adequate prior to the implementation of a population screening programme. However, expanded newborn screening demonstrated that the existing knowledge base for MCADD was inevitably deficient. Prior to population screening, scientific understanding was based on a limited sample of mostly symptomatic patients. Other diseases went through similar transformations, each with its own surprising specificities. Newborn screening for conditions such as carnitine transporter deficiency, for example, led to the identification of maternal disease, calling into question not only previous understandings of the natural history of the disease but also who was the target of screening. At stake in these unexpected findings is the scope of pathology: does a biochemical elevation or a genetic mutation constitute disease in spite of a lack of symptoms?

The genetics staff worked to reassemble what newborn screening undid. Bridging work is aimed at buffering unanticipated consequences produced by the implementation of new technologies. Technologies are implemented with specific objectives but the technologies rarely obtain their goals when implemented and they also generate unintended consequences (Akrich 1992, Timmermans and Berg 2003b). The epistemic component of bridging work implies several interrelated tasks: the recognition of unexpected outcomes, collectively negotiating the parameters of anomalous findings and developing new epistemic characteristics, which in the case of metabolic genetics involves seeking more refined genetic tests and checking observations with colleagues worldwide, as well as formulating new operating procedures to manage the changed understanding of the disease. The continuous tinkering with disease categories affects their ontological status: some diseases split into variants, while others disappeared after being redefined as biochemical oddities without clinical implications. In the case of MCADD, geneticists were able to retain a common disease identity in spite of variations. The geneticists relied on a double move of, firstly, creating a nuanced and diverse understanding of MCADD for diagnostic purposes and secondly, holding on to the traditional treatment regime calibrated for the most severe variant. At worst, the error is harmless overtreatment for MCADD patients.

Although bridging work has a primarily local audience in the clinic, the production of knowledge is situated within a wider knowledge ecology (Star 1995). The geneticists drew upon an international community of experts and their contacts in state laboratories to double check and stimulate scientific knowledge. The knowledge produced in the clinic was only loosely connected to other domains affected by such information. Thus, the testimonies that parents were likely to encounter on the internet before they spoke to the genetic staff reflected pre-screening MCADD fatalities and morbidity (Timmermans and Buchbinder 2010). Parents also felt judged as overreacting when they brought their infants to the emergency department after a prolonged episode of vomiting. Their paediatricians often knew little about MCADD. In those instances, parents needed to bridge a new set of epistemic gaps aimed less at changing the nature of disease than at educating healthcare providers in what MCADD had become.

The extensive ontological redrafting of disease categories in the clinic did not undermine the newborn screening programme. Many factors beyond what happens in the clinic play a role in the institutionalisation of a screening programme but among those factors is that the knowledge produced by clinicians is aimed at making the programme work as intended. Geneticists facing anxious parents felt they had little choice but to work out the anomalous findings because the screening results suggested that a child could be at risk for a preventable metabolic crisis. Not only does the clinicians' ontological bridging work help to sustain the programme's promise to identify metabolic conditions: expanded newborn screening detects and creates metabolic disease.

Acknowledgements

This study was supported by grants from the National Science Foundation (grant SES 0751032) and the UCLA Faculty Senate. We are grateful to John Heritage, Rocio Rosales, Arianna Taboada and the staff and patients of the genetics clinic for their contributions to the research. We also thank the reviewers and guest editors for helpful comments.

Notes

1 C8 is a measure of fatty acids in the blood. Pre-screening, it was considered to be the principal biochemical indicator of MCADD.
2 C2 and C10 measure different fatty acids and hexanoylglycine is an indicator of MCADD in urine.

References

Akrich, M. (1992) The de-scription of technical objects. In Bijker, W. and Law, J. (eds) *Shaping Technology/Building Society: Studies in Sociotechnical Change*. Cambridge: MIT Press.

Andresen, B.S., Dobrowolski, S.F., O'Reilly, L., Muenzer, J., McCandless, S.E., *et al.* (2001) Medium-chain acyl-CoA dehydrogenase (MCAD) mutations identified by MS/MS-based prospective screening of newborns differ from those observed in patients with clinical symptoms: identification and characterization of a new, prevalent mutation that results in mild MCAD deficiency, *American Journal of Human Genetics*, 68, 6, 1408–18.

Armstrong, D. (1979) Child development and medical ontology, *Social Science and Medicine*, 13, 1, 9–12.

Aronowitz, R.A. (2008) Framing disease: an underappreciated mechanism for the social patterning of health, *Social Science and Medicine*, 67, 1, 1–9.

Bowker, G. and Star, S.L. (1999) *Sorting Things Out*. Cambridge: MIT Press.

Buchbinder, M. and Timmermans, S. (2011) Medical technologies and the dream of the perfect newborn, *Medical Anthropology*, 30, 1, 56–80.

Epstein, S. (1996) *Impure Science: AIDS, Activism, and the Politics of Knowledge*. Berkeley: University of California Press.

Greene, J.A. (2007) *Prescribing by Numbers*. Baltimore: Johns Hopkins University Press.

Gregersen, N., Winter, V., Curtis, D., Deufel, T., *et al.* (1993) Medium-chain acyl-CoA dehydrogenase (MCAD) deficiency: the prevalent mutation G985 (K304E) is subject to a strong founder effect from northwestern Europe, *Human Heredity*, 43, 6, 342–50.

Hedgecoe, A. (2004) *The Politics of Personalized Medicine*, Cambridge: Cambridge University Press.

Iafolla, A.K., Thompson, R.J. and Roe, C.R. (1994) Medium-chain acyl-coenzyme A dehydrogenase deficiency: Clinical course in 120 affected children, *Journal of Pediatrics*, 124, 3, 409–15.

Kerr, A. (2005) Understanding genetic disease in a socio-historical context: A case study of cystic fibrosis, *Sociology of Health and Illness*, 27, 7, 873–96.

Kirk, S.A. and Kutchins, H. (1992) *The Selling of the DSM: the Rhetoric of Science in Psychiatry*. Hawthorne: Aldine De Gruyter.

Kuhn, T. (1962) *The Structure of Scientific Revolutions*. Chicago: University of Chicago Press.

Lakoff, A. (2005) *Pharmaceutical Reason: Knowledge and Value in Global Psychiatry*. Cambridge: Cambridge University Press.

Latimer, J., Featherstone, K., Atkinson, P., Clarke, A., *et al.* (2006) Rebirthing the clinic: the interaction of clinical judgment and genetic technology in the production of medical science, *Science, Technology, and Human Values*, 31, 5, 599–630.

Maier, E.M., Liebl, B., Roschinger, W., Nennstiel-Ratzel, U., *et al.* (2005) Population spectrum of ACADM genotypes correlated to biochemical phenotypes in newborn screening for medium-chain acyl-CoA dehydrogenase deficiency, *Human Mutation*, 25, 5, 443–52.

Mol, A. (2002) *The Body Multiple: Ontology in Medical Practice*. Durham: Duke University Press.

Paul, D.B. (1997) The history of newborn phenylketonuria screening in the US. In Holtzman, N.A. and Watson, M.S. (eds) *Promoting Safe and Effective Genetic Testing in the United States: Final Report of the Taskforce on Genetic Testing*. Bethesda, MD: National Institutes of Health.

Rabeharisoa, V. and Bourret, P. (2009) Staging and weighting evidence in biomedicine: comparing clinical practices in cancer genetics and psychiatric genetics, *Social Studies of Science*, 39, 5, 691–715.

Rose, G. (1992) *Strategy of Preventive Medicine*. Oxford: Oxford University Press.

Rosenberg, C.E. (2007) *Our Present Complaint: American Medicine*. Then and Now. Baltimore: Johns Hopkins University Press.

Schutz, A. (1967) *The Phenomenology of the Social World*. Evanston: Northwestern University Press.

Smith, E.H., Thomas, C., McHugh, D., Gavrilov, D., *et al.* (2010) Allelic diversity in MCAD deficiency: the biochemical classification of 54 variants identified during 5 years of ACADM sequencing, *Molecular Genetics and Metabolism*, 100, 3, 241–50.

Star, S.L. (1995) *Ecologies of Knowledge*. Albany: State University of New York Press.

Timmermans, S. and Berg, M. (2003a) *The Gold Standard: The Challenge of Evidence-Based Medicine and Standardization in Health Care*. Philadelphia: Temple University Press.

Timmermans, S. and Berg, M. (2003b) The practice of medical technology, *Sociology of Health and Illness*, 25, Silver Anniversary Issue, 97–114.

Timmermans, S. and Buchbinder, M. (2010) Patients-in-waiting: living between sickness and health in the genomics era, *Journal of Health and Social Behavior*, 51, 4, 408–23.

Timmermans, S. and Tavory, I. (2007) Advancing ethnographic research through grounded theory practice. In Bryant, A. and Charmaz, K. (eds) *Handbook of Grounded Theory*. London: Sage.

Waddell, L., Wiley, V., Capenter, K., Bennetts, B., *et al.* (2006) Medium-chain acyl-COA dehydrogenase deficiency: Genotype-biochemical phenotype correlations, *Molecular Genetics and Metabolism*, 87, 32–9.

Wailoo, K. and Pemberton, K. (2006) *The Troubled Dream of Genetic Medicine*. Baltimore: Johns Hopkins University Press.

Watson, M.S., Lloyd-Puryear, M.A., Mann, M.Y., Ronaldo, P., *et al.* (2006) Newborn screening: toward a uniform screening panel and system, *Genetics in Medicine*, 8, 5, Suppl., 12S–53S.

Wilcken, B. (2010) Fatty acid oxydation disorders: outcome and long-term prognosis, *Journal of Inherited Metabolic Disease*, 33, 5, 501–6.

Wilson, J.M.G. and Jungner, G. (1968) *Principles and Practice of Screening for Disease*. Geneva: WHO.

Yusopov, R., Finegold, D.N., Naylor, E.W., Sahai, I., *et al.* (2010) Sudden death in medium chain acyl-coenzyme A dehydrogenase deficiency (MCADD) despite newborn screening, *Molecular Genetics and Metabolism*, 101, 1, 33–9.

5

Resisting the screening imperative: patienthood, populations and politics in prostate cancer detection technologies for the UK

Alex Faulkner

Introduction

The history of the introduction of mass cancer screening programmes in the UK is beset with controversy, and it is widely acknowledged that some national screening programmes have been introduced largely due to organised patient and citizen advocacy rather than scientific, clinical and epidemiological evidence. The question of whether to introduce mass population screening programmes raises difficult ethical concerns for public health policy and thus for national governments, which in principle seek the strongest possible scientific arguments for such decisions. An array of testing technologies including x-ray, MRI imaging, ultrasound, and a range of biomarkers have been developed in the attempt to identify cancers at a point where curative or remedial medical intervention is possible. The advent of genetic testing and the science of genomics further complicates the issues confronting governance: 'A new generation of tests for cancer could do more harm than good by increasingly diagnosing tumours which may not pose an immediate health risk, according to a leading cancer specialist' (*The Guardian*, 3 April 2007). In this context it is instructive to examine medical conditions for which screening has been actively considered by policy-makers, but *not* – or at least *not yet* – introduced in the form of national screening programmes. Such is the case in the detection of localised prostate cancer.

The prostate is a small gland found only in men, which is important for sexual and reproductive functioning. It produces a unique protein which is the basis of the so-called 'PSA test', a blood test which is analysed in pathology laboratories. Prostate cancer causes one of the highest rates of mortality amongst the cancers, rates of mortality being exceeded only by lung cancer (Cancer Research UK 2009). Nevertheless, it has become a common aphorism within specialist medical and epidemiological communities that 'many more men die *with* prostate cancer than *of* it' (e.g. Neal and Donovan 1998). In other words, the rate of diagnosis is inflated above the rate of symptomatic progression, mainly due to its association with male ageing and the wide-scale identification of minor tumours (Oliver *et al.* 2001). Part of the increased incidence of the disease is undoubtedly due to the upsurge in use of this PSA (prostate-specific antigen) technology over the last 20 years. It is employed globally as a standard aid to diagnosis of localised occurrence of tumours. However, it does not

The Sociology of Medical Screening, First Edition. Edited by Natalie Armstrong and Helen Eborall. Chapters © 2012 The Authors. Book Compilation © 2012 Foundation for the Sociology of Health & Illness / Blackwell Publishing Ltd. Published 2012 by Blackwell Publishing Ltd.

provide a definitive diagnosis. Debate of the appropriate healthcare system response to localised (that is, organ-confined) prostate cancer[1] has been controversial for two decades. Controversy about mass screening for the disease has revolved around three main issues of scientific uncertainty, first, the role of the PSA test; secondly, the inability to predict which diagnosed cancers will progress to be symptomatic and life-threatening; and thirdly, the lack of convincing evidence about the appropriate mode of treatment (Selley *et al.* 1997). The extent of use of the PSA test in the UK, in spite of government policy not to introduce a national screening programme, led some public health commentators to the view that it amounted to 'screening by the back door' (Donovan *et al.* 2001), causing alarm amongst policymakers: 'Use of the PSA test is swamping urology and radiotherapy services, the Government's cancer tsar has admitted' (UK newspaper report 2006). However, increasing dissatisfaction with the predictive and diagnostic performance of the PSA test has been voiced by the medical professions, even amongst its US scientific originators (Stamey *et al.* 2004), and the controversy is now moving into a new phase. This phase is associated with new large-scale scientific studies of the effects of screening and testing, the scientific development of new biomarkers and potentially improved detection tests, and the development of genomics research.

Given this background, the primary aims of this discussion are first, in the context of men's current experience of localised prostate cancer detection, to outline the main dimensions of the controversy and uncertainty over detection and screening in the UK; secondly, to describe the current and emerging scientific knowledge and technologies that are being developed internationally, changing the scope and significance of the detection issue; and thirdly, to analyse how society has responded to (and constructed) the screening issue through actions including the government's sponsoring of scientific medical research, through its governance of prostate cancer detection risks, and through attempts to cope with an influx of international scientific research and detection technologies, and the public and patient expectations to which they give rise.

A number of sociological approaches can be brought to bear in addressing these aims. It almost goes without saying that risk, science and governance are being drawn ever closer together in late modernity. Testing or screening technologies are explicitly concerned with identifying individual and population disease *risk*, and public health and healthcare policymakers consider *governance* regimes for dealing with such risks. At the same time, the appearance of new scientific knowledge and potential tests raises issues of new *expectations* about risks and preventative strategies amongst various populations. Thus the three most relevant conceptual approaches here are in the sociologies of risk, of governance, and of technology expectations. First, it has to be recognised that the influential thought of Michel Foucault is relevant to this field, combining as it does a concern with both risk and governance, and the development of the societal dynamics between them, with its well-known development of the concepts of governmentality and pastoral power applied to understanding the penetration of the state into individual subjectivities (Bunton and Petersen 1997, Foucault 1979). Secondly and alongside this perspective, the sociology of technology governance is seen as important, as it grapples with issues of how governance traditions are re-negotiated as new market conditions emerge (Fox *et al.* 2007), and with the constructive nature of state governance as it legislates for new fields of technological innovation (Faulkner 2009a and 2009b). And thirdly, the understanding of the social innovation processes of technology has been strengthened by the emergence of a sociology of technology expectations, developed around the insight that 'imaginings, expectations and visions' have a constitutive, generative effect in shaping new fields of science or technology, especially at early formative stages (Borup *et al.* 2006). I return to the application and development of these key conceptual, analytic considerations in the discussion section of this essay, after presenting the main features of the evolving technologies, science, perceived risks, expectations and governance of prostate cancer detection.

The account presented here draws on a wide variety of primary and secondary empirical sources, including medical and epidemiological research reports; surveys of the use and interpretation of the prostate cancer blood test; interviews and conversations with healthcare scientists; public domain testimonies of patients; healthcare policy and medical profession documents and position statements; company financial reports; and websites of companies promoting new tests.

The essay proceeds by setting the account in the context of men's current experience of prostate cancer testing in what can still be regarded as the 'PSA era'. This is followed by accounts of the most significant recent scientific and technological developments, and the related cycles of governance reactions, focusing primarily on the UK, and discussion of new international genetics and genomics-based research and emerging tests, and the governance reactions to these.

The dilemma for men

The evidence about men's attitudes to and experiences of being tested for prostate cancer with currently available technologies shows enormous ambivalence. Illustrating this, one summary of interview-based testimonies of men's experiences concluded:

> Some saw it as a routine test, as 'responsible health behaviour'. . . and recommended that other men of their age should consider it, but others emphasised that it is less straightforward than a cholesterol or blood pressure check and that men need to be fully informed and prepared for the consequences if their results are 'abnormal' (DIPEx.org, 2007).

Likewise, one study found that the experience of uncertainty could persist even after a 'normal' test result (Evans *et al.* 2007). One man with symptoms stated that: 'it's a 'maybe' test. Maybe you have maybe you haven't'. Some men found it difficult to understand the message that PSA test results were not necessarily specific to prostate cancer (it can also indicate benign prostate enlargement). In the same vein, a prostate cancer specialist interviewed for a BBC programme noted that 'unfortunately nowadays we're finding a lot of . . . "nice" prostate cancers, and then having to live with the knowledge that we've got them – for 20 or 30 years'. The programme included an account from a man who had had a PSA test with a positive result at age 57. Having joined a scheme of 'active surveillance', rather than therapeutic treatment, the man said that he thought everyone was increasingly 'living with' cancer and that 'we will call it something else'. He concluded that: 'I *have* cancer but I don't *suffer* from it', starkly emphasising the ambiguity and ambivalence in his experience of a citizen self-concept versus patienthood, partly inside and partly outside the biomedical frame: 'I am not a "cancer patient" – but I am a cancer patient' (BBC Radio 4 2006).

This brief overview of men's experience of the current regime of PSA testing indicates the extreme uncertainty surrounding exposure to the risk even of taking the test, and of its potential results and consequences. It is against this background that must be set the burgeoning research examining the effectiveness of screening-based, opportunistic, or other approaches to detecting localised prostate cancer, and the development of new knowledge of its risk factors and an increasing range of tests associated with this knowledge.

Disease testing: the PSA biomarker

The PSA test was developed in the 1980s. It was first used to assist in the monitoring of, and subsequently in the detection of, prostate cancer, being approved as a diagnostic *aid* by the FDA in 1994. UK public health policy during the 1990s resisted calls for the introduction of population screening using it, on the grounds of the poor performance of the test (high proportions of false negatives and especially false positives – leading to unnecessary biopsies and likely overtreatment with high proportions of side-effects including incontinence and impotence), and the lack of convincing evidence about the most appropriate treatment (Selley *et al.* 1997). The 1990s saw a gradual development of an 'evidence-based' policy that has moved from simple resistance to the deployment of the test, to a policy that has encouraged men contemplating the PSA test to undergo a process of 'informed choice', linked to continued policy resistance to introduction of a mass screening programme. Thus, for example, the major professional body active in governance of clinical practice in the field is the British Association of Urological Surgeons (BAUS), which stated in the late 1990s that:

> 'The unthinking use of PSA, especially in elderly men where it causes distress and anxiety, must be prevented. The role of urologists must be to . . . prevent totally inappropriate investigation . . . and to ensure that in other circumstances PSA testing is only carried out after appropriate counselling' (Dearnaley *et al.* 1999).

The governance of national screening programmes in the UK has been shaped powerfully by the National Screening Committee (NSC) since its formation in 1996, in the heyday of the development of evidence-based policy ideology. Particularly notable during the first decade of the 21st century has been the trend for the NSC to shift from a traditional centralist state-based public health policy rationale toward one based more on the principle of 'informed choice', reflecting broader trends. The case of prostate cancer has led this trend, leading to a shift in the state's and the medical profession's apportionment of responsibility for appraising men's risk status via the PSA test. In the UK this was epitomised by the government's introduction of the Prostate Cancer Risk Management Programme (PCRMP), which emphasises an informed choice and counselling policy. The UK Department of Health describes the PCRMP as an 'informed choice *programme*' (my emphasis), distinguished from but nevertheless set alongside the national 'screening programmes' that are now in place for breast cancer, cervical cancer and bowel cancer. In 2005 the government adjusted the tone of its guidance, which now, rather than essentially being intended to dissuade large numbers of men from undergoing PSA testing, acknowledged a 'considerable demand' and emphasised men's *right* to be tested, following counselling and information-giving. This shift, certainly partly a response to lobbying by prostate cancer charities and activists, introduced a new element of a rights-based discourse of entitlement to testing.

There are concerns amongst the healthcare professions about what 'informed choice' can actually mean. For example, a study of general practitioners' (GPs, family practitioners) consultations with asymptomatic men found that some GPs felt that a ten minute consultation, focusing only on the PSA test, would not be sufficient, one GP believing that: 'I don't know if our language has developed enough with patients nor . . . their thoughts. I think . . . they're difficult concepts . . . getting a patient to . . . a position of truly informed decision-making is, is difficult'. The study concluded that GPs discussed with men some of the limitations of the PSA test, such as its poor predictive value and the potentially unpleasant nature of a biopsy, but much less about the potential for identification of indolent cancers and the lack of evidence regarding alternate treatments (Brett *et al.* 2007).

The most important recent developments related to the PSA testing issue concern a set of very large-scale scientific studies of the effects of screening or testing men for prostate cancer, using the PSA test, which were begun in the late 1990s. Two of these clinical trials published final results in the late 2000s; one UK-based trial of treatment preferences and options (*ProtecT*), remains to produce its conclusions.[3] The two highly-publicised studies of PSA-based screening were published in the same issue of the high-prestige *New England Journal of Medicine* in 2009, and appeared to reach conflicting conclusions. The ERSPC (European Randomised Study of Screening for Prostate Cancer) was a pragmatic trial undertaken in eight European countries, studying over 160,000 men offered the PSA test as part of the different countries' regimes. It concluded that a screening programme may be beneficial, decreasing mortality from the disease by up to 20 per cent, but with an associated risk of high over-diagnosis and over-treatment (Schröder *et al.* 2009). The US-based PLCO (Prostate, Lung, Colorectal and Ovarian) Cancer Screening Trial, which included around 77,000 men randomly assigned to either annual screening or usual care, conversely, reported no significant difference in mortality outcomes after 7-10 years follow-up (Andriole *et al.* 2009). The design of both studies has received some criticism on technical grounds (not detailed here). Thus scientific uncertainty persists.

The two studies received a great deal of mass media coverage, and have been considered together in much subsequent commentary. Following their publication, the Chief Medical Officer in England confirmed that men are entitled to have a PSA test free on the NHS (Chief Medical Officer 2009). As a result of the studies, the UK's National Screening Committee was asked by government to review its advice, resulting in a request for independent academic modelling of screening options and analysis of the new trial data. Having requested modelling work 'to look at the costs, benefits and impact on the NHS of screening different age ranges . . .' (once at age 50; or at various intervals in men aged 50 to 74), the committee concluded that a population screening programme could not be supported, the main reasons being: 'prostate specific antigen (PSA) is a poor test for prostate cancer and a more specific and sensitive test is needed'; 'currently we are unable to correctly identify those cancers which will progress and those which are indolent . . .'; and 'the data relating to incidence, prevalence and treatments is poor . . .' (NSC 2010). The committee decided that the option appraisal and data review should be 'shared with relevant stakeholders' both to assess 'what other drivers there are to screen', and 'what other information, or factors need to be taken into account or have not been uncovered'. Subsequently, the NSC reconfirmed its decision to resist mass national screening (BBC mobile 2010).

In summary, scientific uncertainty, deriving from clinical and healthcare trials, continues. This uncertainty is extreme and the psychological and health risks associated with it are increasingly being diffused through society under policies of shared, informed choice and a counselling mode of interaction between health professionals and men. Such a trend diffuses highly ambivalent statuses of patienthood amongst large sections of the male population. Furthermore, we see a shift in the formulation of policy on informed choice toward a rights-based discourse of entitlement. Although the national policy position against a mass screening programme has been confirmed, there have been recent signs that governance actors are considering more closely the possibilities of *targeted* screening programmes in the UK, in spite of remaining concerns about over-diagnosis and over-treatment. National policymaking is encouraging stakeholder participation, in a way that can be seen as seeking legitimation for the policy process.

Disease testing: a genetic biomarker

While the relatively poor diagnostic performance of the PSA test has become increasingly recognised, even by its originators (Stamey *et al.* 2004), a major international scientific effort to find novel biomarkers to improve detection has been undertaken, which has attracted the attention of health technology assessment practitioners (Sutcliffe *et al.* 2009), showing that it has reached the horizon-scanning radar of public health and healthcare policymakers as governance actors. Most of the novel biomarkers remain in the research phase to date, though one in particular merits discussion here because of the publicity that it has generated.

In November 2006, the devolved medical device regulatory assessment regime of the European Union gave a CE mark (Conformité Européen, the 'safety certificate' that allows marketing to consumers across the EU) to a gene-based test to aid in diagnosis. The test is known in Europe as *Progensa PCA*. It is licensed to Californian company Gen-Probe Inc. from a Canadian biotech company, and was launched in the UK also in 2006. Gen-Probe has formed distributor relationships in countries such as Japan, Asia, Israel, and South Africa, indicating the range of their marketing plans. PCA3 is a gene comprising a segment of mRNA located on chromosome 9, which is over-expressed by prostate cancer cells in around 95 per cent of cases. The fully commercialised test is not yet approved for marketing in the United States. Gen-Probe entered into association with a large pharmaceutical company, GlaxoSmithKline, announcing a Phase III clinical trial in 2009, with a view to obtaining FDA approval in due course.

It is claimed that early results suggest PCA3 provides some improvement over PSA in discriminating patients with benign biopsies from those with malignant biopsy results, and may also have value in identifying patients with less aggressive (slower growing, if at all) cancer. The company has constructed ambitious hopes and expectations around the new technology, the CEO of DiagnoCure (the originator of the technology) being quoted as saying: 'We expect this test to . . . be the first gene-based, adjunctive screen for this devastating disease'. The company visions propose that PCA3 could be available as a point-of-care test in five years' time. Rather than being presented as a potential mass screening test, it has been presented primarily as a technology that can be used to reduce unnecessary biopsies, an issue of major concern, as up to 80 per cent of patients with an elevated PSA level may have a negative biopsy.

DiagnoCure, in a financial summary for 2010, highlights the exposure given to trials of the test in the US and Europe at the European Association of Urology annual meeting and the American Urology Association. It reports an increase in revenue in 2010, attributed mostly to sales of the test in Europe. However, in spite of good validation results for the test, the clinical utility is at best still debated, and certainly regarded as not established by the majority of clinicians, and it has so far received limited acceptance both in the US and the UK healthcare systems. The NHS is thus maintaining its cautious 'not yet' resistance to a role for the test. In the UK the National Horizon Scanning Centre produced a brief review of evidence about PCA3 in 2006 (NHSC 2006), but the National Institute for Health and Clinical Excellence (NICE) then rejected it as a topic when it was proposed for a formal Technology Appraisal in March 2007, primarily on the grounds that their review of the initial clinical evidence suggested that it could not distinguish adequately between aggressive and benign tumours (personal communication). Similarly, in the US, the giant health insurance company Blue Cross, on the basis of exhaustive systematic review of the evidence, determined PCA3 and other similar gene-based tests still to be 'investigational' (Blue Cross 2009). At the time of writing, the test is available in a number of private hospitals and centres in the UK. Scientific work continues, for example, with some claims that combined 'multiplex' tests, including additional biomarkers, predict prostate cancer more accurately than any other currently available screening method (Laxman *et al.* 2008).

In summary, gene-expression tests for asymptomatic prostate cancer have reached the attention of centrally important governance actors internationally. Both large insurers and national health technology assessment intermediaries have taken the arrival of these tests seriously enough to examine them with their apparatuses of systematic evidence review and expert committee consideration, and have so far resisted the claims of commercial producers and promoters of the tests. It is notable that in the case of PCA3, the main discourse amongst promoters is one of prevention of unnecessary biopsies (sometimes painful, and costly and not wholly reliable), rather than as a replacement for PSA testing. Gene-expression tests such as these are biomarkers for existing cancer-related abnormalities, in this respect like PSA, rather than predictor tests for a risk of future disease, to which I now turn.

Testing for risk: genome-wide association studies and tests

The final major strand of scientific research comprises the so-called genome-wide association studies (GWAS). The PCA3 and similar tests quantify the extent of gene expression, but do not analyse DNA itself for variations and mutations within genes. As is well known, genome-wide studies have been made possible by the mapping of the human genome, and there is now a massive range of international scientific efforts examining potential associations with prostate cancer. The field is regarded as important enough to have been subject to major review by the US National Cancer Institute (NCI 2010). Some typical case-control studies have been able to identify single nucleotide polymorphisms (SNPs) in different chromosomal regions within a selected population, and, further, combining them have been able to show a good to fair (though debated in significance) association with prostate cancer cases (*e.g.* Zheng *et al.* 2008). Such studies and tests developed from them have attracted the attention of the public health and healthcare governance bodies of the UK and National Health Service. The role of the mass media in representing the results and possible implications of such studies has also been conspicuous, and itself has attracted responses from the central gatekeepers of clinical and healthcare practice.

One set of genome research in particular has caught the media and governance attention in the UK. This is led by scientists at the UK's Institute for Cancer Research and funded by the charity Cancer Research UK, the UK's largest cancer charity. Widely reported, with commentary such as: 'The breakthrough means a new genetic test for prostate cancer could be developed to identify men at high risk who could be targeted for regular screening and early treatment' (*The Independent* 2008), the research identified a number of SNPs with fair association with prostate cancer (Eeles *et al.* 2008, 2009). Research leader Eeles was quoted as saying: 'These findings show genetic medicine is going to happen. We will be starting research this year on developing a genetic test which could be available in three to four years. But we need to ask first who should provide it and how it should be done. It would be irresponsible for a genetic testing company to develop this and sell it over the Web' (*The Independent* 11 February 2008). As part of such a development, Eeles also refers to a new trial just starting in men with a family history of the cancer, to see 'who would come forward, who would benefit, what kind of results do they get on their biopsies and what kind of cancer develops'.

However, in spite of the relatively cautionary stance from scientists, some commercial biotech companies are already making 'direct-to-consumer' tests available. In January 2008, US company Proactive Genomics, a spin-off from Wake Forest university in the US, launched a $300 genetic test, *Focus5*, that examines five SNPs. Icelandic company deCode Genetics announced four more SNPs in November 2009 and linked this finding to the UK-led Eeles' research. They now offer a test stated to identify eight DNA markers, for £250, called *deCODE ProstateCancer*. The company refers to their test as a 'risk prediction' test, or a 'risk test', advising that it is similar in principle to cholesterol level as a predictor of cardiovascular risk. The company promotes expectations about the technology by making a discursive link between 'risk prediction' and current medical services: 'Know your risk and get a complete risk assessment from your physician . . .' (DecodeMe website 2010). Professional counselling is also recommended. Part of the typical vision being promoted is one of empowerment: another direct-to-consumer company, 23andMe, has also developed a test, based on 5 SNPs (23andMe 2010). Their promotional material too emphasises empowerment, while also noting that lifestyle and environment may contribute to prostate cancer risk. Generally, the marketing information does not refer to mortality, the primary outcome in the large PSA screening studies, nor to stage of cancer.

Even though prostate cancer genome-wide association studies have been fruitful, in general they have attracted criticism. Resistance to the adoption of tests has focused espe-cially on their clinical utility. For example, the UK's NHS National Genetics Education and Development Centre, which aims to help promote genetics education to NHS profes-sionals, has evaluated the five gene-variant test published by Zheng and colleagues referred to above, concluding that the clinical utility is less than the PSA test (Li-Wan-Po *et al.* 2010). To find gene variants associated with disease aggression, more large studies, correlat-ing SNPs with disease recurrence and/or mortality rates, are advocated by epidemiologists and public health doctors. In the UK, in particular, the Eeles and other related studies have attracted comment from the NHS's 'National Knowledge Service' (NHS Choices 2008). The commentary on the Eeles study plays down the clinical importance of the findings. Stating that: 'the contribution of each of these genetic variants is modest . . . they explain only about 6% of the familial risk'; 'none of the variants have been proven to affect how these genes function'; 'this study included only men whose prostate cancer was likely to have had a genetic component'; and the study 'included white men from the UK and Australia only' (NHS Choices 2008). Interestingly, this cautious commentary in its explicit 'behind the media headlines' approach refers in detail to the many newspaper reports of the GWAS studies that raised the profile of the screening issue, and thus public expectations, pointing out the 'differing information about the increased risk' that they communicated. However, in spite of these reservations, the National Knowledge Director at the helm of the NHS Choices service concluded that 'there may be a place for a focused screening programme. Research to assess the effectiveness of a screening programme is now needed' (NHS Choices 2008). This raises the prospect of a suite of large screening-related GWAS trials, which could be similar to those discussed above for the PSA test.

In summary, the emergence of genome association studies expands the possibilities for the detection of existing prostate cancer to one of the assessment of potential risk of future disease susceptibility. Some early GWAS-derived tests have been launched, public expecta-tions raised, and visions of future testing countered by evidence-based public health dis-courses formulated through state governance actors. The volume of uptake of the tests emerging in the private healthcare and direct-to-consumer commercial marketplace is unknown, but it is certain that such tests will be further developed and there will be some demand, especially from at-risk populations.

Discussion

Although we are still in the PSA era, the controversial field of localised prostate cancer detection is being expanded by molecular biomarkers and genome-variant associations as tools or potential tools. While confidence in PSA is on the wane, it nevertheless remains deeply embedded, not only in clinical practice, but also in public health policy, and in men's subjective health status, as illustrated in this essay.

It has been necessary to provide detailed accounts of the co-evolution of the science/ technologies of prostate cancer detection and their governance in order to provide the basis for advancing conceptual analysis of this field. The introduction to this analysis noted three strands of theory that are especially germane in approaching issues of the governance of prostate cancer detection: sociologies of risk and governmentality, technology governance, and technology expectations.

In this context, the essay described how the UK governmental 'risk management' policy *diffuses uncertainty* into society and men's subjectivities. This can be regarded as a form of medicalised ambivalence, in which risk associated with 'evidence-based' uncertainty is percolated into men's subjective experience, as shown. Such an interpretation accords with a Foucauldian view of governmentality and pastoral power (Foucault 1979). In the UK, conservative gatekeeping of prostate cancer risk-testing has been re-shaped by a developing acknowledgement of the consequences of what 'informed choice' means in practice via its extension to a recognition of citizens' entitlement – *right* – to be tested if so desired, given an environment of scientific and medical uncertainty. This move represents a further extension of the principle of individual responsibility that was already inscribed into the informed choice policy, in which the state has somewhat relinquished its custodial position over public health, in an acknowledgement that an informed citizen can be also a rights-motivated citizen. This, in turn, can be interpreted as an enhancement of what has been called, in a Foucauldian vein, the 'responsibilisation' of the individual whose health status may (or may not) be at risk (Lemke 2005). Although this concept has been especially applied in terms of an 'imperative of genetic responsibility' where people are seen to harbour risk as potential carriers of disease through families (Hallowell 1999), it is apposite here in understanding the PSA-fuelled UK government risk management policy. Thus, in the case of PSA, responsibilisation has been extended to the state recognition of a right to access precarious metrics of individual disease status. This might be termed a policy of 'informed rights'. Men have become authorised as more 'active citizens' than is implied merely by the informed choice principle. Given that this move is in part a response to lobbying by patients' prostate cancer groups, this can be regarded also as in part a democratic response to the voice of stakeholder interest groups. So at this point the analytic understandings of risk and of technology governance dovetail, highlighting a key dynamic of contemporary technology governance: matters of regulation evolve in uneasy balance with matters of individual responsibility and rights, in which the achievement of societal consent is a negotiated, conflictual, open-ended process under changing environments (*cf.* Fox *et al.* 2007).

In the UK, the policymakers' call for a screening option appraisal suggests that a targeted screening programme, using the 'old technology' of PSA, with carefully-calibrated screening intervals, has not been ruled out. At the same time, the leading national public health policy director (Sir Muir Gray) contemplates the potential of evaluating possible screening using the findings of genomic science – the new technology. As pressures on the NHS to assess the utility of novel molecular biomarkers increase, there are tensions and conflicts in stakeholders' deployment of 'evidence' about these new testing technologies. The institutions of knowledge production, such as Health Technology Assessment, are closely coupled with regulatory agencies such as NICE, national policymaking bodies, and reimbursers. As the account in this essay has shown, in the UK a range of NHS and governmental gatekeepers has shaped the current policy position, ranging from the regulatory decision-making bodies such as NICE and the National Screening Committee, to the rather different *knowledge management* work of the Horizon Scanning Centre, health technology assessment, and the National Knowledge Service. These varying institutions between them form the institutional governance infrastructure constituting the UK's national discourse on prostate cancer detection and screening.

Bearing in mind this governance infrastructure, when we turn to reflect on the emergence of genetic biomarker tests and those derived from genome-association studies, the account above shows that we are moving to different forms of risk and additional, newly-emergent forms of governance. These changes are characterised by visions and expectations of a future risk testing and disease detection marketplace, underpinned by scientific knowledge disputes, and formulated in large part in a mediatised sphere of claim, commentary and counter-claim. The launch of various direct-to-consumer tests in the private, global market-place is integral to this process, and represents a key change in the technology governance environment. Although the genetic biomarkers are to date being positioned by their promoters largely as additional tools in the diagnostic pathway, the concept of *predictive* genome variant-based screening raises a host of social, ethical and legal issues all over the world (*e.g.* Sleeboom-Faulkner 2010). While it is not the place of this essay to elaborate on these, it is notable that we saw in the analysis of the future-looking statements made by scientists and test-developers, that population-level concepts of public health, service design, commissioning, or healthcare system innovation were conspicuously absent. The governance action of healthcare gatekeepers has been an 'evidence-based' resistance to the emerging claims and tests derived from this fast-moving science, a form of governance that accords with the 'lightness of touch' which Fox *et al.* (2007) noted as the mode of contemporary governance of pharmaceutical advertising. In this sense, the governance action here is both traditional and innovative: it has assumed a traditional public health, protective custodian role on behalf of citizens, rather than promoting individual responsibilisation and citizen autonomy but, on the other hand, the mode of governance acknowledges the importance of the media and internet as source of information and expectation for citizens and patients, and thus has intentionally produced an information media-oriented governance response.

As noted, the visions and expectations published in information media by stakeholders are evidently important dimensions of the dynamics of governance of prostate cancer detection. A challenge for the field of the sociology of technology expectations (Borup *et al.* 2006) is to take account of how a range of different actors might contribute to the shaping of pathways of technological innovation, at different points and in different parts of the innovation process. In the case considered here, we observe a lacuna between the emerging knowledge being produced by the sciences of genomics and genetic epidemiology, and the visions of population screening for disease management that are promulgated by some scientists, headline-seeking science journalism and mass media. Thus, there is an arena of informaticised expectations being constructed in the public sphere as part of the discourse of screening and risk around prostate cancer. So far, streams of risk management practice and discourse have focused, on the one hand, primarily on the practical use of the PSA biomarker and, on the other hand, on the genetics and genomics-related promissory science and initial tests, and these streams have remained largely separate. This may change. In the activity of the 'National Knowledge Service', we can see governance work motivated by centralised national public health principles, intervening in a form of *expectations management* that acknowledges the societal importance of mediatised information flows in representing, and arguably distorting, science and technology innovations. This is a more 'upstream' engagement between governance and scientific knowledge, which recognises the powerful promissory component of the representation of scientific findings, illustrating again how a governance tradition is being reconfigured in conjunction with new market conditions (Fox *et al.* 2007). Thus, here we see the strands of theorising on technology expectations and on technology governance drawn together.

Overall in the field of prostate cancer testing and screening, we are witnessing both a multiplication of forms of risk that are becoming testable, and a multiplication of the institutional modes of governance that shape the field. In the era of translational research in medicine, it is easy to assume that the powerful sciences and technologies of genetics and genomics will inevitably find their way into all corners of disease, healthcare and society. In this vein, the public health genomics movement proceeds from a broad assumption that: service issues in public health genomics requiring attention include: 'the integration of genetic and molecular science into mainstream medicine; the evaluation and regulation of genetic tests and complex molecular biomarkers; the . . . evaluation of genetic screening programmes' (PHG Foundation 2010). However, the extent to which such expectations might be, or should be fulfilled, given the governance developments shown here and the resilience of established clinical and social practices using poor-performing but deeply embedded technologies, and the extent to which this might occur across all fields of cancer, let alone other medical conditions, are questions that sociologists of health, science, medicine and healthcare must continue to investigate empirically, and critically.

Notes

1   'Localised' prostate cancer was formerly termed 'early' prostate cancer in clinical discourse, but this has been dropped because it conveys an impression that there will be 'later' development of cancer associated with its initial detection – which is not the case for the majority of cases where the organ-confined disease is detected.
2   DIPEx (Database of Individual and Patient Experience) has grown into a new service, 'healthtalkonline': http://www.healthtalkonline.org. It contains the same material on people's prostate cancer experiences as referred to here.
3   The scientific and social significance of the *ProtecT* trial and its related studies have been discussed in detail elsewhere (Faulkner 2010).

References

23andMe (2010) *About prostate cancer*. https://www.23andme.com/health/Prostate-Cancer/Accessed July 2010.

Andriole, G.L., Crawford, E.D., Grubb, R.L., *et al.* (2009) Mortality results from a randomised prostate-cancer screening trial, *New England Journal of Medicine*, 360, 13, 1310–19.

BBC mobile (2010) *Experts Scrap Prostate Screening Proposal*. http://www.bbc.co.uk/news/health-11930979. 6 December 2010, accessed December 2010.

BBC Radio 4 (2006) *Am I Normal?* Broadcast on 14 November 2006.

Borup, M., Brown, N., Konrad, K. and van Lente, H. (2006) The sociology of expectations in science and technology, *Technology Analysis and Strategic Management*, 18, 3/4, 285–98.

Blue Cross Blue Shield Technology Evaluation Center. (2009) *Special Report: Recent Developments in Prostate Cancer Genetics and Genetic Testing*. http://www.bcbs.com/blueresources/tec/vols/23/special-report-prostatecancer.html. Accessed July 2010.

Bunton, R. and Petersen, A. (eds) (1997) *Foucault, Health and Medicine*. London: Routledge.

Bunton, R. and Petersen, A. (eds) (2005) *Genetic Governance: Health, Risk and Ethics in the Biotech Era*. London and New York: Routledge.

Chief Medical Officer (2009) *Prostate Cancer Screening: Revised Prostate Cancer Risk Management Programme (PCRMP) Information Materials Now Available*. London, Department of Health.

Clements, A., Watson, E., Rai, T., Bukach, C., Shine, B. and Austoker, J. (2007) The PSA testing dilemma: GPs' reports of consultations with asymptomatic men: a qualitative study, *BMC Family Practice*, 25, 8, 35.

Dearnaley, D.P., Kirby, R.S., Kirk, D., Malone, P., Simpson, R.J. and Williams, G. (1999) Diagnosis and management of early prostate cancer, *BJU International*, 83, 18–33.

Donovan, J., Frankel, S., Neal, D. and Hamdy, F. (2001) Screening for prostate cancer in the UK: seems to be creeping in by the back door, *British Medical Journal*, 323,7316, 763–64.

DIPEx (2007) *Prostate Cancer*. http://www.dipex.org. Accessed July 2007.

Eeles, R.A., Kote-Jara, Z., Giles, G.G., *et al.* (2008) Multiple newly identified loci associated with prostate cancer susceptibility, *Nature Genetics*, 40, 316–21. doi:10.1038/ng.90.

Eeles, R.A., Kote-Jarai, Z., Al Olama, A.A., *et al.* (2009) Identification of seven new prostate cancer susceptibility loci through a genome-wide association study, *Nature Genetics*, 41, 1116–21. doi:10.1038/ng.450.

Faulkner, A. (2009a) *Medical Technology into Healthcare and Society: a Sociology of Devices, Innovation and Governance*. Basingstoke: Palgrave Macmillan.

Faulkner, A. (2009b) Regulatory policy as innovation: constructing rules of engagement of a technological zone for tissue engineering in the European Union, *Research Policy*, 38, 4, 637–46.

Faulkner, A. (2010) Trial, trial, trial again: reconstructing the gold standard in the science of prostate cancer detection. In Will, C. and Moreira, T. (eds) *Medical Proofs, Social Experiments: Clinical Trials in Shifting Contexts*. Farnham: Ashgate.

Foucault, M. (1979) Pastoral power and political reason. In Carrette, J.R. (ed.) (1999) *Religion and Culture*. Manchester: Manchester University Press.

Fox, N., Ward, K. and O'Rourke, A. (2007) A sociology of technology governance for the information age: the case of pharmaceuticals, consumer advertising and the Internet, *Sociology*, 40, 2, 315–34.

Hallowell, N. (1999) Doing the right thing: genetic risk and responsibility. In Conrad, P. and Gabe, J. (eds) *Sociological Perspectives on the New Genetics*. Oxford: Blackwell.

Laxman, B., Morris, D.S., Yu, J., Siddiqui, J., *et al.* (2008) A first-generation multiplex biomarker analysis of urine for the early detection of prostate cancer, *Cancer Research*, 68, 645–9.

Lemke, T. (2005) From eugenics to the government of genetic risks. In Bunton, R. and Petersen, A. (eds) *Genetic Governance: Health, Risk and Ethics in the Biotech Era*. London and New York: Routledge.

Li-Wan-Po, A., Farndon, P., Cooley, C. and Lithgow, J. (2010) When Is a genetic test suitable for prime time? Predicting the risk of prostate cancer as a case-example, *Public Health Genomics*, 13, 1, 55–62.

NCI National Cancer Institute (2010) *Polymorphisms and Prostate Cancer Susceptibility*. http://www.cancer.gov/cancertopics/pdq/genetics/prostate/HealthProfessional/page4/. Accessed July 2010.

NHSC National Horizon Scanning Centre (2006) *Prostate Cancer Gene 3 (Progensa PCA3) Assay in the Diagnosis of Prostate cancer*. Birmingham: NHSC, University of Birmingham.

NHS Choices (2008) *Prostate Cancer Genetics*. http://www.nhs.uk/news/2007/Pages/Prostatecancergenetics.aspx. Accessed July 2010.

NSC National Screening Committee (2010) *UK National Screening Committee – Note of the Meeting Held on 16th June 2010*. http://www.screening.nhs.uk/meetings. Accessed July 2010.

Neal, D. and Donovan, J. (1998) Screening for prostate cancer, *Annals of Oncology*, 9, 1289–92.

Oliver, S.E., May, M.T. and Gunnell, D. (2001) International trends in prostate-cancer mortality in the 'PSA era', *International Journal of Cancer*, 92, 893–8.

PHG Foundation (2010) *Foundation for Genomics and Population Health – 'Making Science Work for Health'* http://www.phgfoundation.org/pages/definition.htm Accessed July 2010.

Schröder, F., Hugosson, J., Roobol, M.J., *et al.* (2009) Screening and prostate-cancer mortality in a randomized European study, *New England Journal of Medicine*, 360, 13, 1320–8.

Selley, S., Donovan, J., Faulkner, A., Coast, J. and Gillatt, D. (1997) Diagnosis, management and screening of early localised prostate cancer, *Health Technology Assessment*, 1, 2, whole volume.

Sleeboom-Faulkner, M. (ed.) *Frameworks of Choice: Predictive and Genetic Testing in Asia.* Amsterdam: Amsterdam University Press.

Stamey, T.A., Caldwell, M., McNeal, J.E., Nolley, R., Hemenez, M. and Downs, J. (2004) The prostate specific antigen era in the United States is over for prostate cancer: what happened in the last 20 years? *The Journal of Urology*, 172, 1297–301.

Sutcliffe, P., Hummel, S., Simpson, E., Young, T., Rees, A., Wilkinson, A., *et al.* (2009) Use of classical and novel biomarkers as prognostic risk factors for localised prostate cancer: a systematic review, *Health Technology Assessment*, 13, 5, whole volume.

Zheng, S.L., Sun, J., Wiklund, F., *et al.* (2009) Genetic variants and family history predict prostate cancer similar to prostate-specific antigen, *Clinical Cancer Research*, 15, 1105–11.

6

A molecular monopoly? HPV testing, the Pap smear and the molecularisation of cervical cancer screening in the USA

Stuart Hogarth, Michael M. Hopkins and Victor Rodriguez

Introduction

In 2002 the US diagnostics company Digene was approaching profitability after a decade of work on a molecular alternative to the Pap smear. Their bid to enter the cervical cancer screening market had put Digene in the vanguard of companies developing new genomic diagnostics and their 2002 annual report to investors expressed the company's ambitions thus:

> We expect gene-based diagnostic tests will create a fundamental shift in both the practice of medicine and the economics of the diagnostics industry. Gene-based diagnostic tests will create an increased emphasis on preventative molecular medicine. Physicians will be able to use these tests for the early detection of disease and to treat patients on a personalized basis, allowing them to select the most effective therapy with the fewest negative side effects. Furthermore, companies that develop gene-based diagnostic tests may obtain intellectual property protection and, therefore, may generate higher margins. (Digene 2002: 2)

Digene's vision of the clinical potential of genomic technologies is shared by many scientists, research funders and clinicians, and the genomic turn in the life sciences has generated substantial public and private investment in research for early disease detection (exemplified by the US National Cancer Institute's Early Detection Research Network). However, Digene's commercial vision is not without controversy. In particular, attempts to capture the economic value of genomics through DNA patenting have met with opposition from groups of scientists, clinicians and non-governmental organisations (see Parthasarathy 2007).

Naturally, sociologists are interested in the genomic turn in biomedicine, a phenomenon whose multiple dimensions are captured in the concept of molecularisation. The focus on molecules in biomedical research and clinical practice can be traced back a century (de

The Sociology of Medical Screening, First Edition. Edited by Natalie Armstrong and Helen Eborall.
Chapters © 2012 The Authors. Book Compilation © 2012 Foundation for the Sociology of Health
& Illness / Blackwell Publishing Ltd. Published 2012 by Blackwell Publishing Ltd.

Chadarevian and Kamminga 1998). However, many scholars follow Clarke *et al.* in defining contemporary molecularisation in genomic terms as 'attempts to understand diseases at the (sub)molecular levels of proteins, individual genes, and genomes . . . partially displacing previous emphases on germs, enzymes and biochemical compounds' (Clarke *et al.* 2003: 175, see also Rose 2007: 12). Their view that genomic molecularisation is partially displacing earlier forms of molecularisation is central to our first research question: does the scale and pace of change suggest that the molecularisation of screening is best characterised as a process of revolution or of reform? Much of the hype surrounding genomics suggests the dawning of a new era, but there is good reason to be wary of grand claims: the introduction of new molecular diagnostics has often been resisted and, even when adopted, molecular techniques have often complemented rather than supplanted alternative practices (de Chadarevian and Kamminga 1998). On the other hand, more radical disruption is expected by some, who associate mere accommodation within the 'old value network' as likely to 'kill' the diagnostic innovations (Christensen *et al.* 2009: xxviii) seen as exemplars of a new 'precision medicine' paradigm (Christensen *et al.* 2009: xxii). This article seeks to extend our understanding of molecularisation as a fragile and contested process by characterising its impact on mainstream screening programmes.

Our second research question relates to the commercial dimensions of molecularisation. Digene's 2002 annual report promised commercial gain as well as clinical benefit, predicting 'a fundamental shift in . . . the economics of the diagnostic industry' by allowing companies to achieve 'higher margins' through 'intellectual property protection'. The latter was a reference to Digene's patents on human papilloma virus (HPV) DNA, commercial assets which they used to exclude rivals from the US market. For Clarke *et al.*, gene patents exemplify how genomic molecularisation is interlinked with the 'corporatisation and commodification' of healthcare and biomedical research (Clarke *et al.* 2003: 167, cf. Rajan 2006 on biocapitalism). The commodification of genomic data in the form of gene patents has particular significance for the diagnostics industry, which has traditionally been a high-volume, low-margin business where companies compete on the price and technical quality of their testing platforms (Hogarth 2007). Molecular diagnostics companies like Digene have sought to disrupt this traditional model by using DNA patents to create diagnostic monopolies and thus drive up prices. Such a shift is linked to a change in the R&D process for new tests: instead of being a process involving multiple parties, public and private, a single company plays a more central role, albeit often in collaboration with academic partners (Hogarth 2007). Again, we must be wary of overemphasising the novelty of this trend: de Chadarevian and Kamminga have described how molecularisation has always been engendered through novel configurations of links between industry, the laboratory and the clinic (1998: 1), but many scholars believe that in recent decades the genomic turn in the life sciences has intensified this process; the 'corporatization of the life sciences . . . has simultaneously been rapid and hegemonic on the one hand and contingent and contested on the other' (Rajan 2006: 4). Molecularisation as we conceptualise it here involves not simply the development and diffusion of new DNA diagnostics, but an innovation process quite distinct in its commercial orientation from that of the first generation of cancer screening programmes. Thus, our second research question is: to what extent is the molecularisation of screening engendered through a process of corporatisation linked to new business models in the *in vitro* diagnostics (IVD) industry?

Our choice of case study allows us to build on Casper and Clarke's seminal account of how the Pap test has been 'massaged and manipulated' to transform it into a reasonably 'right' tool' for cervical cancer screening (1998). Their article was an explanation of what we might term the Pap paradox. The test is widely credited with lowering cervical cancer mortality internationally and has been described as 'the most effective screening test for cancer that has ever been devised' (Dehn *et al.* 2007: 2), but with 15–50 per cent false negative rates (that is, the failure to identify cervical cancer when it is present), the Pap has long been problematised as expensive, subjective and error-prone (Cox and Cuzick 2006). The test requires highly trained laboratory personnel (cytologists) who examine cervical epithelial cells by microscope and, while cytology retains its primacy in cervical cancer screening programmes, there have been protracted and expensive attempts to replace or automate the Pap technique (Casper and Clark 1998, Keating and Cambrosio 2003). Digene's DNA-based Hybrid Capture test does not detect cervical cancer but instead identifies specific HPV infections associated with the onset of cervical cancer. This article describes this most sustained challenge to the Pap's long primacy, exploring the dynamics of molecularisation in the context of one of the most established technologies in cancer screening.

Like Casper and Clarke we do not offer a symmetrical account giving equal weight to all actors, but focus on the company that has dominated HPV testing in the USA to provide an account of how market forces play an increasingly central role in screening innovation. Medical screening in the USA is delivered within a complex healthcare system in which the private sector plays the primary role. Delivery of publicly funded health care is increasingly in the hands of for-profit hospitals and 70 per cent of healthcare insurance is privately provided by health insurers, health maintenance organisations (HMO) or preferred provider organisations. This complex institutional architecture shapes screening services in a number of ways. For instance, the search for cost efficiencies has encouraged the growth of a handful of major commercial reference laboratories who collectively deliver a significant portion of clinical testing in the USA, making pathology big business. Cancer screening programmes such as the Pap smear are lucrative commercial markets as they involve large populations that are subject to regular repeat testing, and have facilitated the emergence of novel service configurations, such as the breast care centres which provide mammography and subsequent treatment for women who test positive. It is this highly commercialised testing market which Digene sought to exploit with its new molecular technology.

Building on the prior insights of Clarke and colleagues, this article seeks to make a contribution to the sociology of screening by exploring and extending the concept of molecularisation, delineating how this process unfolds in the context of major screening programmes for cervical cancer in the USA.

Method

Developing a robust history of the first Food and Drug Administration (FDA)-approved test for the detection of HPV required a mixed method historical process study (Van de Ven 2007). Firstly, we undertook exploratory searches of trade and scientific literature and diagnostics industry news websites to reveal key investors and organisations in the HPV field. Additionally, patent literature searches[1] and bibliographic searches aided the detailed mapping of these organisations, their activities and their links. Using these data, 12 interviewees were selected based on their involvement with developments in HPV diagnostics in the USA and the EU, as evidenced by their authorship in major articles, patents and guidelines. Industry executives, clinical scientists, laboratory directors and physicians were interviewed, including supporters of technological options that compete with Digene's kits. We were further informed by numerous additional interviews undertaken to understand the nature of the diagnostics sector as a whole.[2] Semi-structured interviews of 40–150 minutes in length were recorded and fully transcribed. Interviews have well-documented limitations as sources for recent histories (Hughes 1997). In particular social scientists need to be reflexive about interviewees' partisanship and should triangulate data from different sources (Van de Ven 2007). We therefore used the interviews selectively, primarily to identify key themes and events. Triangulation involved using a range of contemporary sources to reach convergent findings. Technical accounts from the scientific literature, statutory filings by companies, patent documents and commercial databases on corporate biotech activities are particularly advantageous as, unlike anonymous interviewees, these are subject to peer reviews, patent examiners or statutory requirements on corporate disclosures. Less rigorous sources such as mainstream and biomedical news articles can still reveal viewpoints and aid chronology. Additionally, we used available scholarly histories (Casper and Clarke 1998, Reynolds and Tansey 2009).

Conceptual approach

Our conceptual framework for charting molecularisation characterises 'technology' as a 'sociotechnical ensemble' (Bijker 1995) of artefacts and techniques embodied in people, and whose operations are structured by a regime of norms, regulations and organisational constraints. This builds on prior categorisations of co-evolving technology components (for example, Fleck 2000) and looks beyond artefacts such as devices or therapeutics that were the focus of much prior work on medical innovation (for example, Blume 1992, Gelijns and Rosenberg 1994, Martin 1999). Embracing alternative approaches such as Keating and Cambrosio's (2003) 'biomedical platforms' and Parthasarathy's (2007) 'medical architectures' we stress the importance of wider institutional and structural influences on technology.

Following previous work (Hopkins 2004, 2006), we adopt Blume's (1992) framework to capture such influences. Here, technological innovation is conceived as occurring through the formation of networks of actors who shape these artefacts, techniques and regimes, according to a shared vision of its future application. As in the social worlds perspective, we reject the notion that non-human actors have as much influence as human actors (Casper and Clarke 1998).

In order to highlight key features of the evolution of HPV testing and screening we utilise four key concepts drawn from Blume's work: *problematisation, inter-organisational links, visions* and the *career*. Blume suggests that technology evolves through a series of problematisations, whereby groups of actors seek to address features of their environment, a technology or its usage that they find problematic. Influential actor groups often occupy a position of power over others in the network and such influence is traceable through inter-organisational links (for example, contracts to provide services, grant provision, formal or informal research collaborations). Influence may also be found in explicit statements of intent to the future shaping and application of technology. These visions (exemplified by the statement from Digene's 2002 annual report above) are an important way of enrolling support by appealing to common objectives. These dynamics of technological innovation can be followed longitudinally using Blume's concept of the career, a sequence of milestones and phases (exploration, development, adoption and growth) that mark the trajectory from bench to widespread practice.

Blume's framework can accommodate insights from a range of related studies and concepts in biomedicine. The central focus on networks and inter-organisational links provides the opportunity to observe processes of entrenchment of new and old technologies in which actors, linkages and visions of technological options become mutually attuned – see Koch and Stemerding's (1994) study of Danish cystic fibrosis screening was molecularised. This helps to reveal actors' difficulties in constructing or re-configuring networks and regimes to accommodate or make acceptable new technological options (Koch and Stemerding 1994). In this article we identify the importance of particular problematisations, organisational links and Digene's vision in each of the four phases of the career of the HPV screening test and use Blume's framework to explore the analytical concepts described above.

The four phases of the HPV test's career

Exploration (1983–1988)

In 1983 Professor Harald zur Hausen's team at the German Cancer Research Centre discovered an association between HPV type 16 infections and cervical cancers. Their viral infection-mediated model of cervical cancer would eventually win zur Hausen a Nobel prize, but it was initially highly controversial. Overcoming this resistance required the opening of new fields of research, in part led by companies seeking to develop new technological options for cancer vaccines and diagnostics (Reynolds and Tansey 2009), including new competition for the Pap test.

During the mid-1980s researchers at laboratory-supplier BRL-Life Technologies (BLT) began work on a commercial HPV test. Local collaborators (researchers, clinicians and pathologists) at Georgetown University provided them with graded cervical cancer samples. Initially BLT's goal was to understand the epidemiology of HPV types 16 and 18 in patients: essential data for the clinical validation of an HPV test. However, they discovered that many of their samples were not infected with these known high-risk HPV types. Thus the researchers, led by Attila Lorincz, turned to identifying novel HPV types, discovering and cloning a number of high-risk strains, while their collaborators at Georgetown made other important discoveries (see Table 1). This work placed Lorincz at the forefront of international research on HPV and cervical cancer, alongside George Roth at the Institut Pasteur in France. Like his French counterparts Lorincz patented his discoveries, something which zur Hausen had not done. This was a move that would prove as important to Digene's future success as Lorincz's growing scientific reputation.

Even at this stage we can see how the commercial development of the HPV test required the creation of inter-organisational links (Blume 1992) enmeshing corporate researchers with academics and clinicians in the established regime of cytology screening. BLT's research in identifying new HPV types demonstrates that the corporatisation of biomedical research undermines any simple model of basic research as an academic function, and the patenting of HPV strains by both BLT and their academic counterparts illustrates how the commercialisation of biomedicine has become entrenched in the practices and values of public institutions.

Development (1988–1999)

In 1988 BLT became the first company to gain FDA approval for an HPV test: the ViraPap kit, composed primarily of synthetic nucleic acid probes. However, despite some clinical uptake, regulatory approval did not lead to commercial success. Many pathologists and cytologists had expressed profound scepticism about the utility of HPV testing, perhaps unsurprising, given that the status of HPV as the cause of cervical cancer remained contested at this time (Reynolds and Tansey 2009). ViraPap also suffered technical limitations: it was radioactive so had a short shelf life, was potentially hazardous to lab staff and it detected only a small number of HPV types (of which many were increasingly being discovered).

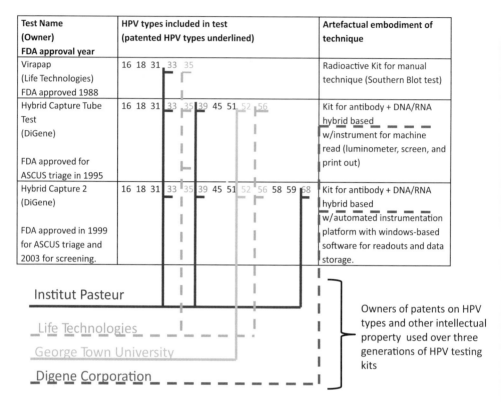

Test Name (Owner) FDA approval year	HPV types included in test (patented HPV types underlined)	Artefactual embodiment of technique
Virapap (Life Technologies) FDA approved 1988	16 18 31 33 35	Radioactive Kit for manual technique (Southern Blot test)
Hybrid Capture Tube Test (DiGene) FDA approved for ASCUS triage in 1995	16 18 31 33 35 39 45 51 52 56	Kit for antibody + DNA/RNA hybrid based w/instrument for machine read (luminometer, screen, and print out)
Hybrid Capture 2 (DiGene) FDA approved in 1999 for ASCUS triage and 2003 for screening.	16 18 31 33 35 39 45 51 52 56 58 59 68	Kit for antibody + DNA/RNA hybrid based w/automated instrumentation platform with windows-based software for readouts and data storage.

Institut Pasteur

Life Technologies

George Town University

Digene Corporation

Owners of patents on HPV types and other intellectual property used over three generations of HPV testing kits

Table 1 *Features of three generations of human papilloma (HPV) test – applications, HPV types, intellectual property, and artefactual embodiment*

In 1990 a frustrated BLT sold their molecular diagnostics division to Digene, a small rival with its own HPV detection technology. ViraPap's failure informed Digene's future strategy which had two elements: technical development and clinical research. While others continued to identify dozens of new HPV types, Digene developed a new detection technique that they named Hybrid Capture (HC). Patented in 1992, this was a non-radioactive method (see Table 1) for detecting specific HPV strains by hybridising HPV DNA from clinical samples with complementary RNA sequences in the kit. Detection of HPV was through antibodies that captured the DNA-RNA hybrids created from an HPV-infected sample. Its key technical advantage was improved sensitivity to HPV strains. Digene's HC test outperformed rivals reliant on widespread techniques that were so sensitive, they even showed positive results to air-exposed swabs that had picked up background particles of the ubiquitous virus (Lorincz *et al.* 1992, Reynolds and Tansey 2009).

Digene hoped their new HC kit would become, in Casper and Clark's terminology (1998), the right tool for HPV testing. ViraPap had failed, in large part because of clinical reluctance to adopt HPV testing, so clinical adoption of Digene's new proprietary technology required consensus on what job it should be doing in cervical cancer screening programmes:

We thought that a molecular determination of the virus that causes cervical cancer could minimally provide additional new information to the cytologists and the

Table 2 *Three possible roles for human papilloma virus (HPV) testing in cervical cancer screening*

Testing protocol	Description	Molecular status
ASC-US triage (reflex)	Pap remains initial screening test, HPV is used as a reflex follow-up, reducing need for colposcopy	Secondary
Adjunctive screen with pap	Pap and HPV used as joint primary screen allowing less frequent screening for women who test negative for both tests.	Equal
Sole primary screening test	HPV used as initial screening test, Pap is used to follow-up HPV-positive women.	Primary

Source: Developed by authors from primary material. ASC-US, atypical squamous cells of undetermined significance; Pap, Papanicolaou smear.

pathologists to help them improve the quality of the Pap smear, but we had it in the back of our mind that maybe the Pap smear was not as great as it had been claimed, and that . . . we might be able to find a superior method, either a more sensitive or more specific or more prognostic in some way. So yes, that was, that was in our minds all right: that the Pap smear was competition. (Digene executive)

From the outset Digene's clinical vision for the molecularisation of cervical cancer screening centred on a problematisation of the Pap test and the promotion of HPV testing as a solution to the limitations of the entrenched technology, but they were uncertain whether molecularisation would entail supplanting or merely supplementing the Pap test. Table 2 illustrates the range of options, ranging from a secondary to a primary role for the HPV test. Addressing this uncertainty was the second element in Digene's strategy and pursuit of this goal required Digene to broaden their network and make significant financial investment in clinical trials.

During the 1990s Digene invested in multiple large head-to-head clinical studies against the Pap test, in a series of collaborations with charities, government departments, universities and research institutes across the world. By 2003 Digene had participated in HPV tests involving 'an aggregate of approximately 90,000 women on four continents' (Digene 2002: 12) and had increased their annual R&D expenditure to $10,262,000. This made Digene the primary sponsor and shaper of HPV clinical trials, placing them at the centre of a global research network, as illustrated by Figure 1, which shows links with key scientific collaborators (that is, those they produced four or more co-authored articles with). The strong inter-organisational links with the National Cancer Institute (NCI), Johns Hopkins and the HMO Kaiser Permanente, are particularly clear.

Digene collaborated with Kaiser Permanente and NCI on two studies crucial to adoption of the HC2 test for use in the triage of patients with atypical squamous cells of undetermined significance (ASC-US: see Table 2). Digene gained FDA approval for use of the HC2 test in ASC-US triage in 1999. This suggests that, at this stage in the career of their technology, Digene was taking a cautious approach to the molecularisation of cervical cancer screening

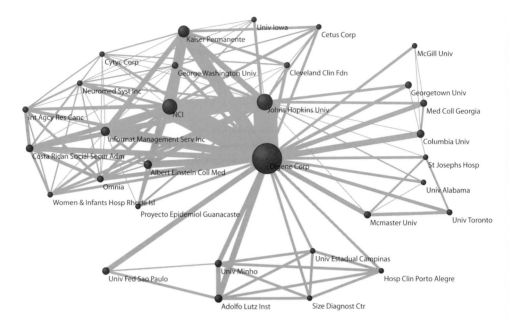

Figure 1 *Digene Corporation's main co-authorship links (by affiliation) on scientific papers*
Source: Thomson-Reuters' Web of Science publications data for 'Digene' in author address. Node size
relates to the number of papers co-authored with Digene (only shown for N > 4). Line size is proportional
to the number of publications co-authored by the two organisations lines connect. Layout based on
Kamada-Kawai algorithm using Pajek freeware with no weighting for line similarity.

in the US market, seeking to support rather than supplant the Pap test's status as the entrenched gold standard. FDA approval marks the end of the development phase for Digene's HC2 test.

Adoption 1999–2003
This period saw Digene's HC2 test become entrenched in cervical screening in the USA. By 2003 Digene had gained key customers, such as the major reference laboratories, giving them 62 per cent of the ASC-US triage market and the company had finally become profitable. Pivotal to adoption was data from the NCI-funded ASC-US/LSIL Triage Study for Cervical Cancer (ALTS) trial, for which Digene provided supplies free of charge. Data from this trial were crucial for the inclusion of HPV testing in clinical guidelines by the American Society for Colposcopy and Cervical Pathology (ASCCP):

> It [the ALTS trial] validated the performance of the test in predicting CIN 3. It was such a widespread study and the recommendations based on that through ASCCP pretty much directed the growth of that test (US LAB 2).

The 2001 guidelines state that (providing a suitable sample was collected with the initial Pap test) clinical data from multiple studies had proved that HPV testing was a better way of triaging women with ASC-US than traditional options of repeat cytology or immediate colposcopy. The justification for the recommendation shows that the test was valued for the ease with which it could be added to the existing cytology-based screening process:

[W]omen do not need an additional clinical examination for specimen collection, and 40% to 60% of women will be spared a colposcopic examination. Moreover, women testing negative for HPV DNA can rapidly be assured that that they do not have a significant lesion. (Wright *et al.* 2002)

Further support came in 2002 in guidelines issued by the American Cancer Society (ACS).

Digene now had a growing clinical evidence base, externally validated through peer review, FDA approval and endorsement in clinical guidelines. To speed adoption of their test, Digene made large investments in sales and marketing. The traditional marketing route for diagnostic companies is to enrol the support of laboratory directors who then promote new tests to physicians. However, Digene employed a dedicated sales force directly targeting physicians, a strategy seen by some investors as essential to drive rapid adoption of new molecular diagnostics [personal communication with US venture capitalist], and observed in other genetic test developers, such as Athena and Myriad Genetics. (Secretary's Advisory Committee on Genetics Health and Society 2010).

The extent of Digene's network is illustrated by the ASCCP and ACS guidelines. Amongst the 41 members of the ASCCP working groups who contributed to the guidelines, there were seven individuals disclosing links with Digene, ranging from study grants to honoraria and consultancy work. Similarly, five of the 38 working group members for the ACS guidelines disclosed some link to Digene. Both guidelines stated that only studies using the HC2 test had been taken into account when assessing the utility of HPV testing, indicating the extent to which Digene's R&D investment had given it a dominant position in the HPV-testing research network.

Growth (2003 to the present)
Following the adoption of the test for triage, Digene focused on the larger primary screening market (see Table 2), while their growing sales and the market entry of other companies signalled a widespread validation of the molecular approach to cervical cancer screening. Use of Digene's test for triage of ASC-US cases was the low-hanging fruit of HPV testing. It exploited a chief clinical problematisation of Pap testing, namely, the large number of ambiguous results requiring further follow-up, but did not challenge Pap's status as the gold standard. It was, moreover, a relatively small market. Perhaps unsurprisingly, most of Digene's R&D investment was focused on the more lucrative primary screening market, funding studies where HPV testing was a routine adjunctive screen alongside the Pap test or an alternative to it. In 2002 guidelines from the ACS recommended HPV testing as an adjunctive screen in women over 30 years of age (again, citing only studies funded by Digene) and in 2003 this indication gained FDA approval. The advantage claimed for the combined screening technologies was that women with negative results need not be tested again for three years (in the USA, annual Pap testing was the standard of care). The HC2 was renamed DNAwithPap, an indication of Digene's vision of a future where the molecular and the cytological were inextricably linked. Long-time Digene collaborators Kaiser Permanente were early adopters, again demonstrating the importance of key inter-organisational links (such as the research collaborations indicated in Figure 1), but also illustrating the significance of institutional structures in building early adoption:

The Kaiser Permanente HMO model was ideally suited in some ways to making such a drastic change. First, because Kaiser directly cares for its paying members, it did not have to convince outside payors to cover the additional test. Second Kaiser employs its physicians, so if the administration wanted to add a new laboratory test, it could do so without formal buy-in, though implementing the test requires the understanding and cooperation of the ob/gyn providers. (Southwick 2004)

Elsewhere, however, clinician adoption of this screening protocol was slow. Compliance with the new guidance required physicians to forgo annual examinations with patients who tested negative with Pap and HPV tests (Southwick 2003), thus challenging what one pathologist described as 'the strongly ingrained emphasis on annual Pap smear screening' (Stoler 2001). Digene responded by adopting a new marketing strategy: direct-to-consumer advertising. When Digene's advertising campaign launched, the media reported public and professional disquiet. Among those quoted in the media was Dr Alan Waxman, co-author of the American College of Obstetricians and Gynecologists (ACOG 2003) guidelines, and a sceptic about adjunctive HPV screening:

> It's another way of screening . . . But to recommend it would give it higher priority over the Pap alone, and I don't think the data is there to support that. (Rosenwald 2005)

A molecular monopoly: protecting market share

Despite such clinical resistance the HPV market has grown rapidly. Most insurance companies cover HPV testing; it is mandated by a number of states such as California and Maryland and it is available through the public Medicaid system in most states. Industry estimates suggest that more than 10 million tests are performed annually and that the market has grown 40 per cent in each of the past 5 years. However, not all HPV testing is done using Digene products. A 2006 survey suggested that other tests were being used in 19.1 per cent of US labs, either alongside Digene's HC2 test or instead of it (Moriarty et al. 2008). Testing labs were developing their own tests from scratch or using component reagents sold by companies such as Ventana and Third Wave. Digene sought to restrict such competition by using its intellectual property rights and the FDA regulatory regime as barriers to market entry.

Digene had a legal monopoly through the right to exclude others from commercialising tests on the high-risk HPV strains they had patented or licensed for diagnostic use in the USA (see Table 2). Between 2001 and 2009 Digene defended their dominant patent position in a series of US law suits with rivals Gen-Probe, Roche, Beckman Coulter and Third Wave. Digene further reinforced their proprietary defences through a strategy of technological autarky. Many molecular diagnostics companies focus on producing reagents that can be run on other companies' platforms but Digene chose to create its own self-contained instrumentation system to ensure they were not dependent on potential rivals: 'we didn't want to be subject to the vagaries of the other company who was at any moment going to be our competitor' (Digene executive).

Digene exploited their status as the only company with an FDA-approved test clinically validated in multiple large studies as an additional way to try and protect its market hegemony: 'Digene set the bar very high and FDA have kept it high' (US industry executive). This argument was set out in an editorial which accompanied the ACSSP's 2001 guidelines: '[The] bar has been raised for bringing forward newer HPV diagnostics . . . Any new test must document its performance relative to this standard' (Stoler 2002: 2140). In 2006 new ACSSP guidelines went further, suggesting that less well validated tests 'may increase the potential for patient harm' (Wright *et al.* 2007). These statements illustrate how Digene's test had become the gold standard for HPV testing.

Controversy about the use of tests that have not been approved by FDA was aired in 2005 in an article in *CAP Today*, the magazine of the College of American Pathologists. The article quoted Digene's NCI collaborator, Marc Schiffman:

> I do not want to see decades of careful research lessened in their impact by sloppy application or sloppy thinking. If a well-meaning laboratory applies an HPV test that doesn't work right, then a beneficial technology has just been made malignant.

Also commenting was Lorincz, Digene's CSO: 'We spent tens of millions of dollars validating this test. For someone to come along and run 70 or 80 patients verges on the insult to everybody' (Titus 2005). In 2007 the issue was raised again, this time in an article in *Clinical Laboratory News*, a magazine published by the American Association for Clinical Chemistry (Levenson 2007).

Digene's dual strategy was largely successful in excluding rivals in the US market but it was ultimately unable to prevent Third Wave from launching an FDA-approved test, ending Digene's near decade as monopolist. However, by this time Digene had been bought for $1.6 billion by the Dutch company Qiagen. The acquisition price demonstrated the perceived value of the market for Digene's HPV test (and thus the commercial success of their strategy) because the company had little in its development pipeline (Baker 2006).

Yet, for HPV-testing sceptics, the scale of this acquisition simply confirmed that cervical cancer screening was under threat from the forces of commercialism. In a lengthy 2008 editorial defending the role of cytology, the pathologist R. Marshall Austin sounded the alarm:

> No one observing the changing field of cervical cancer screening could now reasonably overlook the multi-billion dollar financial interest just behind the scenes, nor industry's close affiliations with scientific thought leaders and organizations. (Marshall Austin 2008)

The article presented cytotechnologsts as the guardians of quality cervical cancer screening and urged the continuation of education programmes for cytologists. Despite such clinical resistance, commercial interest continues to be fuelled by Digene's vision of a molecular HPV test to replace cytology:

> All the players in the market are betting on the transition to a model where all women get the [HPV] test first. This would increase the size of the market by tenfold. (US industry executive).

The enduring power of Digene's vision continues to be sustained by their R&D investment and the network of collaborations it spawned, such as the UK-based 'HPV in Addition to Routine Testing' trial, whose findings were published in *The Lancet*, where Cuzick argued that Digene's test could be used as the sole primary screen, with Pap testing relegated to a secondary role as a follow-up test for HPV-positive women (Cuzick *et al.* 2003). By 2006 some US pathologists were suggesting that the end of Pap testing was in sight: 'New studies and current data suggest that with increasing sensitivities, we may see women moving from the HPV test in combination with Pap to the HPV screen alone' (Borgert 2006). For now, such predictions remain visionary statements which suggest that the molecularisation of cervical cancer screening is a process that has yet to run its course.

Discussion

Given the huge levels of public and private investment in genomic research, increasing numbers of molecular screening technologies are likely to enter clinical practice in coming decades. It is therefore important to gain a clear understanding of the social dynamics of innovation in this field. We have sought to answer two key questions: does the scale and pace of change suggest that the molecularisation of screening is best characterised as a process of revolution or of reform, and to what extent is the molecularisation of screening engendered through a process of corporatisation linked to new business models in the IVD industry? Our history of HPV testing has used Blume's established conceptual framework for tracking the co-evolution of the networks, artefacts, techniques and regimes. This conceptual lens has allowed us to extend the utility of the sociological concept of molecularisation in the context of cancer screening.

HPV testing has been available for nearly 20 years and is the most commonly used molecular technology for cancer screening, but it has failed to supplant the Pap test. Instead the molecularisation of cervical cancer screening has required an accommodation with cytology. This reflects the wider picture in oncology, where diagnosis still relies on the morphological examination of tumour biopsies. This evolutionary model would appear to be consistent with the broader history of diagnostic innovation in the 20th century: 'The newer modes of analysis have not necessarily replaced the older ones. In many ways, the history of these techniques has been one of continuous accretion' (Amsterdamska and Hiddinga 2003: 426). This mirrors the uptake of biotechnology in pharmaceutical R&D processes, where new biotechnological techniques were used to re-invigorate traditional small molecule drug discovery as well as supporting the development of novel biological therapies (Hopkins *et al.* 2007). As the historian David Edgerton has suggested, we should not mistake the first appearance of a technology for its triumphant dominance, and older technologies may be increasing in use, even as new ones are growing in popularity (Edgerton 2006: 31–2).

Our account of the Pap's persistence as the gold standard for cervical cancer screening supports Bowker and Star's (1999) contention that established standards have significant momentum and may endure over long periods of time because they span multiple communities of practice (in this case, cervical cytologists and obstetricians or gynaecologists). However when problematised, they may be opened up, but the new practice must also submit to the growing need in the era of evidence-based medicine for multiple forms of standards (Timmermans and Berg 2003). This would appear to be a key site of contestation in the molecularisation of screening. Molecular diagnostics companies like Digene present their products as inherently more standardised and standardisable than older techniques but their success in challenging established standards will be contingent on multiple factors.

How, then, should we characterise the process of molecularisation? Clarke *et al.* (2003: 184) suggest that technoscientific innovations in biomedicine are cumulative and do not immediately replace older alternatives but that nevertheless they 'tend to drive out the old over time'. Keating and Cambrosio state that 'in the era of "molecular pathology" one might be tempted to say that biology has supplanted pathology as the form of explanation of disease' (2003: 331) but they also suggest that, at the level of specific technologies, biomedical innovation may be about supplementing rather than supplanting: 'new platforms are often articulated and aligned in complex ways with existing ones, and thus integrated into an expanding set of clinical-biological strategies' (2003: 4). Our case exemplifies this dynamic of entrenchment through integration; the addition of HPV to established testing protocols can be understood as simply the latest chapter in the story set out by Casper and Clarke (1998) of how successive forms of tinkering were necessary to ensure that Pap testing remains the right tool for the job.

Our second research question concerned the relationship between molecularisation and commodification and corporatisation. The history of laboratory diagnostics in the 20th century was one of professionalisation and the creation of new sub-disciplines such as microbiology and radiology. The Pap smear exemplified that trend, predicated as it was on the creation of a new cadre of cytology specialists (Casper and Clarke 1998). The promotion of Pap testing was largely carried out by non-profit organisations such as the ACS (Casper and Clarke 1998). By contrast, HPV testing exemplifies a new trend: the increasing importance of diagnostic companies in the development and diffusion of innovative molecular diagnostics.

Digene's enrolment strategies involved a dynamic process of deepening engagement. In the first place it suited clinical researchers to collaborate with Digene, who might either subsidise or pay for clinical trials. Secondly, as early data demonstrated the robustness of their test, it gained credibility as a dependable research tool whose use in multiple trials across the globe could be expected to produce reliable standardised data that could be subject to cross-comparison and meta-analysis. Finally, as the research community began to produce findings that indicated a possible role for HPV testing in cervical cancer screening, these researchers became advocates for the clinical use of the HC2 technology as the only HPV test which had proved its value in multiple large clinical trials. Digene thus harnessed a growing interest in the clinical potential of HPV testing to create an international research network focused on demonstrating the specific utility of their proprietary HC technology. Digene's problematisation of the research agenda conflated the utility of HPV testing and the utility of their HC test, and thus allowed them to become an obligatory point of passage (Callon 1986) for clinical research on HPV testing.

The success of Digene's problematisation required not only a critique of the Pap test but the establishment of their proprietary technology as the tool of choice for detecting the presence of HPV. This was not simply a question of which company had the most reliable, accurate or convenient technology but also a matter of intellectual property rights, closely related to Digene's commercial vision of higher profit margins from patent-protected diagnostics. Digene's success was achieved not only by enrolling key supporters to drive clinical adoption; but also by excluding competitors from joining the network.

Their strategy's success relied in large part on Digene's scientific reputation for research on HPV and cervical cancer. However, the company's substantial investment in clinical trials was equally important. This case study illustrates how a young, relatively small diagnostic company can become the orchestrator of global networks involving research scientists, funding agencies, laboratory directors, clinicians, patients and regulatory agencies. This is a new 'systems integration' role for diagnostics companies, mirroring that seen in pharmaceutical firms (Hopkins *et al*. 2007), illustrating how molecularisation involves not simply a greater role for industry but a shift in business models. Crucial aspects of Digene's commercial strategy – patenting biomarkers such as HPV DNA to try and gain a period of market exclusivity: marketing direct to physicians, direct-to-consumer advertising, investing heavily in studies to demonstrate the clinical utility of a test – were all relatively novel to the IVD industry. For critics, the strength of Digene's network and its direct-to-consumer marketing strategy were sources of concern. For their supporters, they demonstrated that the company were trying to do the right thing: investing heavily in clinical trials to explore the utility of HPV testing and helping to raise awareness of the benefits of a validated technology that could help save women's lives. Again, we see how collaboration was facilitated by a shared vision that aligned Digene's private interests with the wider public interest.

However, the novelty of the commercial drivers should not deflect attention from the continuities with the Pap story. Public bodies played a pivotal role in the promotion of Pap testing (Casper and Clarke 1998) and were also central to the clinical adoption of the HPV test, especially the NCI who funded the ALTS trial and (alongside the ACS) then championed Digene's HC2 technology as the only robustly validated HPV test. Collaboration with industry has thus reinforced the authority of the established network of public sector actors in US cancer screening.

Conclusion

The molecularisation of cervical cancer screening remains highly contested by sceptics doubtful of its clinical utility and wary of its commercial orientation. As Austin's 2008 editorial indicates, their critique is also a defence of the traditional authority of the medical profession as the arbiters of clinical truth and the guardians of patient care. Austin formulated an alternative problematisation to frame the Pap-HPV debate, suggesting that more was at stake than competing claims for the diagnostic accuracy of rival technologies, instead arguing that 'much of the (U.S.) physician–patient relationship is built on the regular Pap test visit' (Austin 2008: 156). The Pap screen is more than a test; it is a ritual clinical encounter which forms a cornerstone of women s health maintenance regimes. By presenting the HPV test as a fundamental threat both to the effectiveness of those regimes and to the stability of the doctor-patient relationship, Austin indicates not only how contested the molecularisation of cervical cancer screening is, but also how contingent it may be on accommodation with the established medical order and the entrenched technologies that currently underpin it.

The HPV-Pap story brings into question Keating and Cambrosio's assertion that we are now in the 'era of molecular pathology'. It would appear that in cancer pathology it is the microscope, not the microarray, that still holds sway. Our case study suggests that the molecularisation of screening may not be a zero-sum game in which new technologies eventually triumph over old ones; instead, the adoption of novel genomic diagnostics may simply deepen the entrenchment of their older rivals. We have seen the same dynamic at work in the relation to the corporatisation of diagnostic innovation. For all the novel commercial elements in the development process, the entrenchment of the HC2 test in screening protocols required Digene to enmesh itself in the pre-existing network of public actors, in particular the NCI and the ACS, who had worked for decades to establish the Pap smear as the right tool for cervical cancer screening. Thus, just as adoption of HPV testing has reinforced the primary importance of cytology in cervical cancer screening, so too the corporatisation of diagnostic innovation has reinforced the central role of public bodies in the development and adoption of new screening technologies.

Further research is required to understand how generalisable our findings may be. The molecularisation of screening is likely to have a different dynamic in cases where there is no well-established alternative to new genomic technologies. More broadly, we might also wish to compare the molecularisation of screening with molecularisation in other diagnostic applications, such as pharmacogenetics and prognosis. We may find that corporatisation has become even more important in areas outside screening, which, for all its commercial potential, remains a public health priority in which the state and other public sector actors play a primary role.

Acknowledgements

The authors thank the following people: the interviewees who participated; the European Commission's Institute for Prospective Studies (IPTS) who funded this research; the IPTS staff who managed the project – Dolores Ibarreta and Danieli Paci; the project advisory board: Nele Berthels, KU Leuven, Birgit Verbeure, KU Leuven, Kathleen Liddell, University of Cambridge, Eleni Zika (UK Medical Research Council and Belgium European Research Council), and Ismael Rafols for assistance with Pajek.

Notes

1   The study required a full 'patent landscape' to be generated to reveal commercially active organi-
    sations. See Hunt *et al.* (2007) for a description of patent search methods.
2   This work was undertaken as part of an international comparative study of the impact of patent-
    ing on diagnostics, sponsored by the European Commission's Joint Research Centre, IPTS, in
    2008–2009. The study drew on more than 70 interviews in the EU and USA covering aspects of
    patenting in relation to diagnostic innovation and focusing on specific case studies. The HPV
    case study presented here is based on research available in the second and third of the project's
    three peer reviewed reports. These reports are available at http://www.sussex.ac.uk/spru/research/
    kplib/ archives/eteps-ip-pgx (last accessed 22 September 2011).

References

Amsterdamska, O. and Hiddinga, A. (2003) The analyzed body. In Cooter, R. and Pickstone, J. (eds) *Companion to Medicine in the Twentieth Century*. London: Routledge.

Baker, M. (2006) New Wave diagnostics, *Nature Biotechnology*, 24, 8, 931–8.

Bijker, W.E. (1995) *Of Bicycles, Bakelites and Bulbs: Towards a Theory of Sociotechnical Change*. Cambridge: MIT Press.

Blume, S. (1992) *Insight and Industry: on the Dynamics of Technological Change in Medicine*. Cambridge: MIT Press.

Borgert, N. (2006) Testing providers work to improve cervical cancer diagnostics, *Clinical Lab Products*, available at http://www.clpmag.com/issues/articles/2006–10_07.asp (last accessed 18 September 2011).

Bowker, G. and Star, S. (1999) *Sorting Things Out: Classification and its Consequences*. Cambridge: MIT press.

Callon, M. (1986) Elements of a sociology of translation: domestication of the scallops and the fisher-men of St Brieuc Bay. In Law, J. (ed.) *Power, Action and Belief: a New Sociology of Knowledge?* London: Routledge.

Casper, M. and Clarke, E. (1998) Making the Pap smear into the 'right tool' for the job: cervical cancer screening in the USA, circa 1940–1995, *Social Studies of Science*, 28, 2–3, 255–90.

de Chadarevian, S. and Kamminga, H. (eds) (1998) *Molecularizing Biology and Medicine: New Practices and Alliances, 1910s–1970s*. Amsterdam: Harwood.

Christensen, C.M., Grossman, J.H. and Hwang, J. (2009) *The Innovator's Prescription*. New York: McGraw Hill.

Clarke, A.E., Shim, J.K., Mamo, L., Fosket, J.R., *et al.* (2003) Biomedicalization: technoscientific transformation of health, illness, and US biomedicine, *American Sociological Review*, 682161–94.

Cox, T. and Cuzick, J. (2006) HPV DNA testing in cervical cancer screening: from evidence to policies, *Gynecologic Oncology*, 103, 1, 8–11.

Cuzick, J., Szarewski, A., Cubie, H., Hulman, G., *et al.* (2003) Management of women who test positive for high-risk types of human papillomavirus: the HART study, *The Lancet*, 362, 9399, 1871–76.

Dehn, D., Torkko, K.C. and Shroyer, K.R. (2007) Human papillomavirus testing and molecular markers of cervical dysplasia and carcinoma, *Cancer*, 111, 1, 1–14.

Digene (2002) Annual Report, available at http://marketbrief.com/dige/10k/annual-report/2002/9/30/4393963/filing (last accessed 18 September 2011).

Edgerton, D. (2006) *The Shock of the Old: Technology and Global History since 1900*. London: Profile Books.

Fleck, J. (2000) Artefact-activity: the co-evolution of artefacts, knowledge and organisation in technological innovation. In Ziman, J. (ed.) *Technology as an Evolutionary Process*. Oxford: Oxford University Press.

Gelijns, A. and Rosenberg, N. (1994) The dynamics of technological change in medicine, *Health Affairs*, 13, 3, 28–46.

Hogarth, S. (2007) *The Clinical Application of Molecular Diagnostic Technologies – a Review of the Regulatory and Policy Issues*. Report for Health Canada. Cambridge: University of Cambridge.

Hopkins, M. (2004) Technique-led technological change and the hidden research system: genetic testing services in the NHS. PhD thesis, SPRU, University of Sussex.

Hopkins, M. (2006) The hidden research system: the evolution of cytogenetic testing in the National Health Service, *Science as Culture*, 15, 3, 253–76.

Hopkins, M., Martin, P., Nightingale, P., Kraft, A., *et al.* (2007) The myth of the biotech revolution: an assessment of technological, clinical and organisational change, *Research Policy*, 36, 4, 566–89.

Hughes, J. (1997). Whigs, prigs, and politics: problems in the historiography of contemporary science. In Soderqvest, T. (ed.) *The Historiography of Science and Technology*. Amsterdam, Harwood.

Hunt, D., Nguyen, L. and Rodgers, M. (2007) *Patent Searching; Tools & Techniques*. Hoboken: John Wiley and Sons.

Keating, P. and Cambrosio, A. (2003) *Biomedical Platforms: Realigning the Normal and the Pathological in Late-Twentieth-Century Medicine*. Cambridge: MIT Press.

Koch, L. and Stemerding, D. (1994) The sociology of entrenchment: a cystic fibrosis test for everyone, *Social Science & Medicine*, 39, 9, 1211–20.

Levenson, D. (2007) New HPV test brings challenges, *Clinical Laboratory News*, 3361.

Lorincz, A.T., Reid, R., Bennett Jenson, A., Greenberg, M.D., *et al.* (1992) Human papillomavirus infection of the cervix: relative risk associations of 15 common anogenital types, *Obstetrics and Gynecology*, 79, 3, 328–37.

Marshall Austin, R. (2008) Dismantling of the U.S. cytotechnology educational infrastructure is premature and carries significant risks, *Archives of Pathology & Laboratory Medicine*, 132, 2, 154–158.

Martin, P. (1999) Genes as drugs: the social shaping of genetherapy and the reconstruction of genetic disease, *Sociology of Health & Illness*, 21, 5, 517–38.

Moriarty, A., Schwartz, M.R., Eversole, G., Means, M., *et al.* (2008) Human papillomavirus testing and reporting rates: practices of participants in CAP's interlaboratory comparison program in gynecologic cytology in 2006, *Archives of Pathology & Laboratory Medicine*, 132, 8, 1290–4.

Parthasarathy, S. (2007) *Building Genetic Medicine: Breast Cancer, Technology, and the Comparative Politics of Health Care*. Cambridge: MIT Press.

Rajan, K (2006) *Biocapital: the Constitution of Postgenomic Life*. Durham, NC: Duke University Press.

Reynolds, L.A. and Tansey, E.M. (eds) (2009) *History of Cervical Cancer and the Role of the Human Papillomavirus, 1960–2000*, Wellcome Trust Witness Seminar Series. GC/253/A/38. London: University College London.

Rose, N. (2007) *The Politics of Life Itself: Biomedicine, Power and Subjectivity in the Twenty-First Century*. Princeton: Princeton University Press.

Rosenwald, M. (2005) Digene's ads take their case to women, Washington Post, 21 March, accessed online at http://www.washingtonpost.com/wp-dyn/articles/A52466-2005Mar20.html.

Secretary's Advisory Committee on Genetics Health and Society, National Institutes of Health (2010) *Report on Gene Patents and Licensing Practices and Their Impact on Patient Access to Genetic Tests*. Washington: SACGH.

Southwick, K. (2004) Kaiser roll: the push for more HPV screening, *CAP Today*, July.

Stoler, M. (2001) HPV for cervical cancer screening: is the era of the molecular Pap smear upon us? *Journal of Histochemistry and Cytochemistry*, 49, 9, 1197–8.

Stoler, M. (2002) New Bethesda terminology and evidence-based management for cervical cytology findings, *JAMA*, 287, 16, 2140–1.

Timmermans, S. and Berg, M. (2003) *The Gold Standard*. Philadelphia: Temple University Press.

Titus, K. (2005) Making a valid point about HPV tests, *CAP Today*, September.

Van de Ven, A.H. (2007) *Engaged Scholarship*. Oxford: Oxford University Press.

Wright, T., Cox, J.T., Massad, L.S., Twiggs, L.B., *et al.* (2002) 2001 consensus guidelines for the management of women with cervical cytological abnormalities, *JAMA*, 287, 16, 2120–9.

Wright, T., Massad, L.S., Dunton, C.J., Spitzer, M., *et al.* (2007) 2006 Consensus guidelines for the management of women with abnormal cervical cancer screening tests, *American Journal of Obstetrics & Gynecology*, 197, 4, 346–55.

7

Blind spots and adverse conditions of care: screening migrants for tuberculosis in France and Germany
Janina Kehr

Introduction

Tuberculosis (TB) is an infectious disease and until quite recently it was thought that it had been eradicated in France and Germany. The advent of effective antibiotic therapies after World War II and improved living conditions had resulted in declining rates of TB since the 1950s, and the incidence of the so-called 'white plague' had been reduced to manageable proportions by the 1960s and 1970s. As a result, state-controlled screening through chest radiography, which had constituted one of the bases of the French and German national TB control programmes in the post-war years, was widely abandoned (Ferlinz 1996). However, radiography screening did not disappear altogether and in the 1990s was targeted at 'high risk' groups, notably immigrants (Broekmans et al. 2002).[1] In the 1990s immigrants had been shown to have a relatively higher incidence of TB than the the the indigenous population. The response was a policy of active and targeted screening on a European level (Comité national d'élaboration du programme de lutte contre la tuberculose 2007, Diel 2007, Rieder et al. 1994). Thus, having historically been considered a 'social disease' associated with poverty (Barnes 1995, Dubos and Dubos 1987), TB was now thought of as an immigrants' disease, both in epidemiology (Antoine and Che 2010, Brodhun et al. 2007) and in public discourse (Ho 2004, Kehr 2009, 2010, King 2003).

Most social science studies examining the TB screening of migrants focus on their construction as a high-risk group, thus showing that targeted TB screening is not politically innocent but directly linked to national politics, and in particular to the politics of (border) control (Bashford 2010, Craig 2007, Ho 2004, King 2003). These works contribute to the literature on the surveillance and control of at-risk groups through preventive public health measures (Brown 2000, Lupton 1999, Petersen and Lupton 1996). Analysing the discourses of immigration and the nation-state they describe the way public health policies construct different categories of risk, arguing that these categories justify enhanced interventionism and surveillance of migrants, revealing risk to be a central mechanism. It thus comes as no surprise that in these studies, the branding of migrants as being at high risk is found to have stigmatising and politically exclusionary effects. It serves to strengthen state surveillance

The Sociology of Medical Screening, First Edition. Edited by Natalie Armstrong and Helen Eborall.
Chapters © 2012 The Authors. Book Compilation © 2012 Foundation for the Sociology of Health & Illness / Blackwell Publishing Ltd. Published 2012 by Blackwell Publishing Ltd.

through public health arguments – a feature also reflected in historiographic studies carried out on the link between public health, immigration and infectious disease (Coker 2004, Keane and Gushulak 2001, Welshman and Bashford 2006).

One important contribution of these studies is to analyse the concrete aspects of medicine as a surveillance system. Compulsory screening of migrants for TB at entry comes as a pertinent example, as a direct connection between immigration policies, health regulations and population control exists. Yet these studies rely largely on discourse and document analysis to demonstrate their findings and do not sufficiently engage with the whole array of screening practices, which are not always compulsory and are not always directly linked with immigration policies. Very little attention is therefore paid to the practical problems, ambivalences and national differences that arise when migrants are targeted and screened. One exception is the work of John Welshman (2000, 2010) who examines targeted TB screening from a practical perspective. He describes migrant at-entry screening in England and Wales in the 1950s and 1960s. Welshman (2000) shows how a higher incidence of TB among immigrants has led to their surveillance through disease control measures like screening. Yet his study also shows that the screening surveillance system did not operate effectively in practice. Practical problems were faced by public health professionals during screening, such as a failure to organise follow-up care or linguistic and administrative difficulties in attempting to X-ray large numbers of migrants. This limited the actual impact of surveillance and control on migrants, and also the efficiency of diagnosis, thereby partially impeding migrants' early treatment for TB. Welshman's study thus partly contradicts the surveillance thesis proposed by most sociological studies on migrants as an at-risk group, showing its limitations and adverse effects.

Following the historical work of Welshman, my comparative study proposes to continue this line of research into the practicalities, differences and ambivalences of migrant screening. It takes the example of active TB screening in France and Germany, where no social science research has been conducted on this topic to date. Active TB screening, operationalised through chest X-rays, targets at-risk groups or legally defined groups either forcibly, as is the case for at-entry screening of migrants and workplace screenings or voluntarily. Rather than assuming that migrant screening is a problem *per se*, I ask: How do national disease surveillance data actually construct migrants as a high-risk group? How do high-risk group definitions influence (or not) local migrant screening practices and what other factors codetermine the way screening is operationalised? In the case of Roma and undocumented migrants, what political and medical problems arise following screening for TB?

I argue that the main issues for French and German TB screening today are about concrete politics and practices, which cannot be sufficiently taken into account by discourse analyses focusing on risk-constructions and surveillance medicine.[2] I thereby try to overturn the theoretical discussion about screening and surveillance of migrants as an at-risk group by arguing: firstly, that it is not only the stigmatisation of migrants through risk discourse that is at stake in France and Germany, but also the problem of not seeing the most vulnerable among them through crude disease surveillance data; secondly, that the practice of active screening for extremely vulnerable migrants is still an exception in both countries, yet for different reasons; and thirdly, that it is not the way that health risk is used in immigration discourses and politics that is most dangerous for migrants in France and Germany, where TB is neither a reason to be expelled nor a reason to have a residence permit refused. What is dangerous is the way in which restrictive immigration policies interfere with and subvert the voluntary preventive public health activities targeting them, creating difficulties in their early treatment and follow-up care. In arguing thus, the aim of my article is to promote a pragmatic sociology of screening that pays attention to the practical complexities, political conditions and medical ambivalences of screening and care, especially when the groups concerned are socially, politically and medically vulnerable.

The study

The present article is based on research undertaken for my PhD thesis on the contemporary fight against TB in France and Germany, for which I conducted ethnographic fieldwork from 2005 to 2010 in TB prevention centres of two major French and German cities. Through a multi-sited ethnography (Marcus 1995) I 'followed' TB as an object into multiple medical sites, in order to understand by comparison how TB is treated in practice by health professionals today: medically, socially, sanitarily and politically. My research is based on a combination of observation, interviews and the study of documents produced by the actors of the social worlds I studied (Pope 2005, Savage 2000) – working documents, guidelines, articles and standard forms. The study draws on more than 300 hours of annotated observation of the daily activities of TB prevention centres in France ($N > 200$) and Germany ($N > 100$) and informal conversations with doctors, nurses, social workers and public health officers, as well as 23 in-depth interviews with public health professionals (doctors, $N = 8$; nurses, $N = 5$; public health officers and programme managers, $N = 8$; and social workers, $N = 2$). All conversations, interviews and field notes cited in this article were held or taken either in French or in German and translated by the author.

I was admitted to the German TB prevention centre as an intern with the local public health administration. Access to the French TB prevention centres was obtained through direct telephone contact with the responsible public health officers, granting me permission to do research in the departmental public health centres. My identity as an anthropologist and my research objectives were disclosed from the beginning to all actors in both countries, in written as well as oral form, and I obtained permission to observe consultations. I bound myself to respect medical confidentiality. One patient declined my presence. My observations focused on verbatim interactions between health professionals and patients, on collegial conversations, on the practices of health professionals and on the material settings of the sites. Detailed notes were taken where possible and subsequently transcribed. The topics of the semi-structured interviews were identified from preliminary analyses of observational transcripts. They dealt with the practical as well as political and ethical problems of TB control and medical treatment, as identified by the health professionals. I thus not only observed the practices of the health professionals but also listened to them 'as if they were their own ethnographers' (Mol 2001: 15).

I analysed my data comparatively, using each national case to inform the analysis of the other. Following grounded theory (Glaser and Strauss 1967), my research questions were adapted to the study context (public health/France or Germany/professionals or patients) and refined as I carried out ethnography and analysis. I made comparisons not in an entirely symmetrical way but heuristically to elucidate blind spots and to problematise common assumptions (Nader 1994). To do so, I first set the ethnographic data in their respective national contexts. After having identified the main issues through summarising, organising and coding the data, I compared the emerging topics and concepts transnationally. I was thus able to flesh out national particularities or binational commonalities on the one hand, and to localise or internationalise the results of the analysis on the other if the national frames were not sufficient for interpretation. In the present article, a slight dominance of the French data, where I did quantitatively more research, exists.

Migrant screening: from the construction of risk to paradoxes of practice

In the 1970s TB was nearly eradicated in western European countries. But at the end of the 1980s disease rates began to stagnate or to increase again and what had become an almost invisible infection made a re-appearance on public health agendas. A European-wide TB 'task force' was set-up, known as the 'Wolfheze Workshop' (Antoine 2006), whose history has been recently described (Veen *et al.* 2011). One of the main goals of the guidelines following the workshops was to strengthen disease surveillance at national levels, as well as the targeted screening of migrants, 'based on mandatory . . . reports to identify population segments' (Veen *et al.* 2011, table I) at risk.

Blind spots: on bureaucratic disease surveillance and migrant patients
In France and Germany, at-risk migrant groups are primarily defined through annual, nationwide disease surveillance reports based on so-called 'mandatory declarations'.[3] These declarations are transmitted to the disease surveillance institutions for each TB case detected. The definition of at-risk groups thus depends on the epidemiological data available through the declarations and on the way in which epidemiological data are collected and produced. Besides clinical and bacteriological information on the TB cases, the mandatory declarations collect 'key variables' such as age, sex and country of birth, which are processed in the annual surveillance reports. In line with European guidelines, the explicit objective of the French and German annual reports is to elucidate disease risks in different population segments, in order to participate in 'meaningful and effective planning of prevention programmes' (Brodhun *et al.* 2007). Yet despite this aim, the annual surveillance reports based on mandatory declarations in both countries remain remarkably silent regarding TB control programmes and the development of migrant screening strategies.

In Germany, the mandatory declaration is generally very poor with regard to social information on declared TB cases, and particularly regarding key migrant data, like the person's legal status, housing situation or date of immigration. The German declaration only collects information on the patient's country of birth and a revision of the mandatory declaration is – to my knowledge – not scheduled. This inattention to the social situation of TB patients in general and migrants' living conditions in particular is in part due to a broader societal blindness regarding inequalities in health and the specific problems migrants seeking healthcare might face, an issue that was publicly debated in Germany only in the 2000s (David 2001) – contrary to France, where the issue of social rights for migrants has been much debated since the 1970s (Mbaye 2009: 14). This is even more true for undocumented migrants, who have been absent from much public discourse and official statistics in Germany for a long time (Huschke 2011: 157), the health sector included, whereas French social movements early on put undocumented migrants' situation at centre stage in immigration debates (Mbaye 2009: 14). One very practical effect of the socio-political invisibility of undocumented migrants in the German public sphere is that preventive measures targeting them specifically, such as active TB screening, are discussed neither on a political nor practical level (Diel *et al.* 2004). Another effect is that that neither German disease surveillance reports nor public health policies recommend the screening of undocumented migrants – a fact that is accentuated through the legalistic working practice of German public TB control, as I show below.

As one might expect, the situation is slightly different in France, one of the oldest European immigration countries. In the French context, the mandatory declaration is slightly more robust with regard to data collected about migrants' situations. There has been some recent debate around these mandatory reports and a working group has been set up to render them more socially meaningful in informing public health policies. In addition, a 2004 French Ministry of Health working group on preventive TB activities resulted in an expert report specifying how to target particular migrant populations. In the last five years, the mandatory reports have thus come to include some data on the living situation of migrants, such as their housing situation and their date of arrival in France. Data on the diagnostic context have also been collected since 2010, specifying whether diagnosis occurred because the patient was seeking healthcare or due to contact tracing or at-entry screening. Yet there are still very few social facts collected in the French declarations, such as the social security status of migrant patients or their legal status. Thus, annual epidemiological reports lack information on the precise social situation that migrants face when falling ill, which have considerable influence on their disease risk and healthcare trajectories. Data on the diagnostic context are now collected in France and might help to elucidate the healthcare trajectories of different groups of migrant patients and this is thus a first step to educate policymakers on the (in)efficiency of some screening measures for migrants, such as at-entry screening. Yet, to be socially and practically meaningful, these data would need to be read with reference to information concerning migrant patients' social and legal situation – data which are politically and ethically sensitive to obtain and which have until now been collected in neither France nor in Germany.

Knowledge of living conditions of migrants and of the way that these conditions might influence the migrants' risk of disease remains very thin in both countries. This is cause for concern, as social and legal statuses are known to have a strong impact on susceptibility to TB (Antoine 2006, King 2003) and access to treatment (Borde and David 2003, Carde *et al.* 2002). When it comes to the development of targeted screening policies of population subgroups most at risk for disease, the national surveillance reports are therefore insufficient to inform public health practice, despite their political mission to do so. Rewritten in the same format with very similar expressions every year, the German and French surveillance reports based on mandatory declarations are, I would argue, a bureaucratic form of epidemiology but not an effective and practical means to inform prevention programmes, as their mission statements hold.

As Lyle Fearnley (2010) shows in his article 'Epidemic Intelligence', on Alexander Langmuir's concept of disease surveillance, disease reports were conceptualised after World War II to 'provide a continuous picture of the actual extent of an epidemic. Rather than providing the material for causal determinations, the disease report only enabled a "continuous watchfulness" ' (Fearnley 2010: 42) for the state. Relying on mandatory declarations, the annual TB reports bureaucratically fulfil the function of disease monitoring in French and German national spaces today. Yet, contrary to certain forms of epidemiology, be it the 'moral' epidemiology of Virchow or Villermin in the 19th century or the social epidemiology of today (Krieger 2001, Lang *et al.* 2009), surveillance epidemiology is not greatly invested in correlating patterns of social life or living environment with the fact that certain sub-populations fall ill more often than others (Fearnley 2010). Politically 'neutral' state surveillance reports register the amount of disease within a national territory, yet they do not and cannot inform on ways to act on it, remaining silent about the underlying causes of disease – be they social or political. Disease surveillance reports based on socially thin mandatory declarations remain silent about the distribution of TB, which is dissimilar among differently positioned migrant groups in society. The reports therefore struggle with important blind spots. As a consequence, those people most likely to be at risk for TB today – undocumented migrants and those without access to the healthcare system – remain invisible.

Legalism and local know-how: differences in active screening
In the German case, the absence of differentiated epidemiological knowledge on migrants at risk comes with strictly legalistic TB control. Active screening for TB in Germany is mandated by a public health law, the *Infektionsschutzgesetz* that is readily applied in the everyday work of TB prevention centres. This law commissions public TB centres – a branch of the local public health authority – to take chest X-rays of high-risk persons who are legally defined through residential criteria. People so defined include asylum seekers and refugees obliged to stay in a migrants' shelter until a residence permit is granted, homeless people asking for a place in a shelter, and people admitted to an old people's home. In short, those targeted are people residing in collective housing schemes as defined by a public health law.

This legalistic working mode is well demonstrated in a standard phrase I heard repeatedly from TB prevention centre doctors and social workers: 'We work according to the disease control law' the health professionals told me. All the German public health professionals I encountered confirmed that they approach their work purely on the basis of the law. The legal regulation did not leave any room for questions, for example, whether the screening of migrants in keeping with the law was sufficient for disease control and treatment success – questions that did come up in the French context, as I will show later on. Being legally codified, the German screening approach with criteria based on collective residence was, for the doctors and social workers of the German prevention centre, not open to question. They thus screened asylum seekers, refugees, displaced persons and homeless people applying for space in a shelter on a regular basis. Yet neither practical, ethical nor political questions concerning the targeting of specific groups, such as undocumented migrants, were asked in the German field. In effect, even if all migrants from high-incidence countries are defined as a high-risk group, and even if a large German epidemiological study could show that undocumented migrants are particularly at risk for disease (Hauer *et al.* 2006), there is no particular screening practice to target them if they do not belong to the administrative category of asylum seekers and displaced people (Diel *et al.* 2004). As a practical consequence, there is a complete absence of outreach screening of particularly vulnerable migrants.

This is not quite the case in France, where outreach screening is heavily debated in the field. French public health professionals – nurses, programme managers and doctors alike – critique first and foremost the absence of precise data in relation to different migrant groups, as well as the absence of guidelines. During an interview, a public health nurse working in a French centre for TB control reflected on this absence in voicing his uncertainty regarding the groups he works with on a daily basis:

> Do we really reach, well, let's say it this way: which, in fact, are all the types of populations which are most at risk? Do we really reach them? Are we really in contact with them? I am thinking, for example, of the Roma camp where we will be going . . . Because, you know, tuberculosis exists mainly in these places, in disadvantaged neighbourhoods, and people from these neighbourhoods do not necessarily come into the prevention centre to see us. (Nurse, interview, France)

As can be seen through the nurse's words, the translation of group risk into active outreach screening comes with questions and uncertainty. The public health nurse I interviewed in 2005 asked himself whether he really *knew* the groups he should address and he wondered whether he was looking for TB in the right places, whether he could reach out to those who seemed to him to be most at risk. The general, statistical knowledge about at-risk groups, as established by epidemiological surveys and national guidelines that go unquestioned in the German field, were not meaningful enough. In the French context, the general knowledge of at-risk groups in the national guidelines turned out to be insufficient to inform the nurse's practice in the field and did not represent the different groups of people he interacted with in his everyday work.

The responses of a programme manager of a regional TB screening programme in France set up in 2010, that I will call 'PrO-S-TB' (preventive outreach screening for TB),[4] who worked in the same region as the nurse I had interviewed, are also intriguing. We talked about the origins of the PrO-S-TB, which was set up in collaboration with a local non-governmental organisation to reach extremely vulnerable migrants, like the Roma or undocumented migrants in overpopulated shelters. In the middle of our discussion the programme manager, seeming troubled, suddenly said:

> You see, we found 12 TB cases for 300 X-rays identified within PrO-S-TB, this is huge, isn't it? The problem is, we don't have any comparative numbers, so we don't really know whether we should enlarge the circle of people we are targeting. We think that we are going in the right direction, but we don't really have good indications. There are the general guidelines, but not a lot more. (Programme manager, conversation, France)

The statements of the nurse and the programme manager display a sense of uncertainty and unease concerning the targeted screening activities realised by the public health department. Health professionals explain their unease by the absence of meaningful guidelines – an unease that did not exist in Germany where a strong public health law overshadowed possible doubts. Yet the daily practice of the French public health professionals shows that despite this insecurity, they had pursued outreach screening activities targeting vulnerable migrants for many years, resulting in establishment of PrO-S-TB in 2010.

The implementation of PrO-S-TB on a local level demonstrates that the French public health professionals did not rely only on official risk-group knowledge in their daily practice or objectified, 'indisputable' knowledge (Desrosieres 2000). It was much too inaccurate for them. Nor did they rely on a general law, as was the case in Germany. They produced and used for their daily interactions with migrant groups what a public health doctor, in an interview we held about PrO-S-TB, named empirical knowledge (*savoir empirique*) or know-how. To my question as to why they chose to screen migrant shelters as one priority in the programme, the doctor replied:

> It is about our experience . . . We have over 60 migrant shelters in the region. This is a huge number. From our experience in the field, we are acquainted with the living conditions in the shelters. If you count people actually living in a room with eight beds, you will be coming up with a number of 24. We simply know that the situation there is very problematic. (Public health officer, interview, France)

As the different quotations show, empirical knowledge, or know-how, about divergent TB risks among different migrant groups and their living conditions does exist in the field. The local working practice relying on know-how and experience thus partly steps in for the insufficiencies and inaccuracies of the French national disease surveillance data and recommendations. Yet this politically sensitive and complex empirical knowledge remains local and screening thus largely depends on initiatives by engaged health professionals, which are often politically and ethically motivated. One effect of this contingency is that, in most places in France, vulnerable migrants are not systematically screened. In consequence, their TB is often diagnosed symptomatically at a very advanced stage (Bouchaud 2009). A programme like PrO-S-TB, seeking to reach out to vulnerable migrants, remains a localised exception.

As shown earlier, classificatory blind spots in bureaucratic disease surveillance and thus the vagueness and lack of specificity in the definition of at-risk groups make it difficult to develop meaningful and efficient screening activities for vulnerable migrants. In the French context, this situation exacerbates the rarity of active screening programmes, which are dependent on the engagement of public health professionals locally and thus are realised only in exceptional cases. In Germany, the very rigid, legalistic framework, which is out of step with migratory reality and its social dynamics, hinders local initiatives and accounts for the simple absence of targeted outreach screening for some migrant groups, like undocumented migrants. In Germany, such vulnerable migrants not only fall through the statistics in disease surveillance data but they also fall through the screening net, as defined and operationalised by law. Despite the different reasons for the relative absence of active screening for vulnerable migrants, the effects are comparable in both countries: screening approaches to vulnerable migrants continue to be 'suboptimal' (Hargreaves et al. 2009: 140). Yet even more is at stake, as I show in the last section using the example of PrO-S-TB and Roma patients in France. Once an exceptional, local screening programme started to function, it resulted in a tragic situation that depended for the most part on larger national immigration politics that created adverse conditions of care.

Public humanitarianism in France: on exceptional screening practice and adverse conditions of care
The French immigration authorities implemented active screening of migrants in the form of 'at-entry' screening following World War II (Wluczka 2007). Since then, a medical exam including a chest X-ray has become obligatory for all immigrants from non-European Union countries entering France legally for more than three months and is subject to significant fees. Yet as I have shown, undocumented migrants are not captured by this strategy, either statistically or practically. To this end, the French National Programme to Fight Tuberculosis has recommended the active screening of particularly vulnerable migrants in 2007, like undocumented migrants, but also those residing in overpopulated shelters or those with an ambiguous residential status like the Roma. Nevertheless, such screening programmes are barely realised in France. The screening programme PrO-S-TB, which I discuss in more detail, is thus rather exceptional in both senses of the word: exceptional, because the targeted screening of undocumented migrants and Roma is not commonly practised in France; and exceptional because the PrO-S-TB relies on humanitarian, and thus exceptional, conditions of care-giving (Ticktin 2006).

PrO-S-TB is a pilot screening project put in place by an allocation the Ministry of Health accorded to the local public health administration where I did my research. It was set up after a series of highly contagious TB cases were discovered in the region, together with a worrying stagnation of the local disease rates. Two screening activities were established. One consists of screening the inhabitants of migrant shelters using a mobile X-ray unit. The other activity, to be discussed, consists of a collaboration of the public health department with a local charitable health centre, and screens patients without health insurance arriving at the health centre. In practice, most of their patients are undocumented migrants and Roma.

At a public conference presenting PrO-S-TB, the doctor working in the charitable health centre talked about the reasons for the collaboration between public and humanitarian institutions:

> Why should we actively screen for tuberculosis in our health centre? Because our patients' social profiles comprise many conditions for tuberculosis. Our patients are migrants from high incidence countries and they suffer from extreme poverty, poor health, identity controls and everyday harassment. For years we have longed for the active TB screening of our patients, but we could not come up with a solution. And then the miracle in 2010: the local department of public health proposed a collaboration. (Activist doctor, conference transcript, France)

What the activist doctor was enthusing about was the implementation of PrO-S-TB in collaboration with the local public health administration. In practice, the public health department positions a mobile X-ray unit behind the organisation's charitable health centre. Twice a month, the centre's patients – 'people whose living conditions one cannot even imagine', as the responsible public health officer put it (conference transcript, France) – thus get the opportunity to have a free lung X-ray on site.

With this measure, the public TB control unit attempts to reach extremely vulnerable migrants excluded from the public healthcare system and at-entry screening, by screening them at the place where they actually seek and get care, the charitable health centre. As such, the collaboration between a humanitarian organisation and the local public health department can be seen as a form of public humanitarianism for the sections of the population the French state usually does not care for and does not care about. Unpublished data, collected by the public health office, indicate that the screening yield for active TB by PrO-S-TB in the health centre is huge: out of 363 X-rays taken in 2010, 13 TB cases were detected, 11 of which were bacteriologically confirmed. Statistically, this is a yield of 35.8 TB cases per thousand screened (local statistics, conference transcript, France). For comparison: the median yield of immigrant screening in Europe at entry is 2.83 per thousand, as a recent meta-analysis shows (Arshad *et al.* 2010). Comparing these figures to the local data, even accounting for statistical imprecision, shows that at-entry screening is more than ten times smaller than the outreach screening of undocumented migrants by PrO-S-TB at the health centre. The juxtaposition of these numbers shows that the screening of excluded and vulnerable groups through a local public-humanitarian programme, set up with the help of local knowledge regarding their care-seeking trajectories and living conditions, seems a success – at least on a diagnostic level.

Nevertheless, an important question has not yet been asked: what happens to those persons diagnosed with TB? Are they actually treated? The programme manager explained to me that they had made 'good progress on the question of care' (Programme manager, conversation transcript, France). She told me that at the beginning of the programme, they did not even consider that treatment could be a problem. But rapidly they realised that in order to treat patients with TB they had to set up a proper system of assistance so that the patients would actually be hospitalised and treated. The assistance scheme includes translators throughout the hospitalisation process, social workers and community mediators. Yet, once the assistance was functioning and the patients started free treatment, another problem emerged, first and foremost in regard to the medical care of the Roma: treatment completion. Only one in eight treated Roma patients is known to have actually completed it (local statistics, conference transcript, France). This fact led the public health officer and the clinician to ask whether it was a good idea to put Roma patients in treatment in the first place;

a question they answered negatively in some cases. Given the danger of multi- resistance when treatment is abandoned early, as well as the possible severe side effects for the patient in the absence of medical supervision, the public health doctor jointly with the clinician took an ethically painful medical decision: to abstain from treatment for those of their Roma patients who are not in a life-threatening condition.

How can it be that public health doctors and clinicians jointly agree not to treat a patient suffering from a treatable disease? The reasons are political rather than ethical, as the explanations of the public health doctor on the reasons for treatment failure show: she told me that at the inception of the programme there was a political consensus among immigration and public health administrations not to deport Roma patients in treatment and to maintain residential rights for those communities living in the same camp as the person diagnosed with TB. Yet the immigration authorities did not honour the agreement and so some treated patients or their family members were obliged to leave the French territory. Patients thus had to leave the country within a few weeks and were unable to complete treatment in France. In her explanation, the doctor clearly explained that interruption of treatment was not the Roma patients' fault. On the contrary, treatment interruption was seen as a logical effect of restrictive immigration policies in regard to Roma communities. Treatment completion was thus seen as a political impossibility and – in consequence – to begin treatment was to act irresponsibly in medical terms.

The example reveals that it is very much the political discrimination of the Roma that impedes their treatment completion, and thus hinders their continuous care from screening to diagnosis and treatment, a fact of which public health professionals are well aware. The example, furthermore, shows that an apparent preventive solution to high TB incidence – a screening programme with a huge diagnostic yield – has had paradoxical effects. It was adapted to a particular group of vulnerable migrants and was effective in identifying new TB cases. But despite diagnostic efficiency, the strategy turned out to have serious adverse effects for public health and individual care, namely, the possible creation of multi-resistance to treatment and thus the decision to withhold antibiotic treatment from people who are most vulnerable to disease. This last ethnographic example of practice shows that tackling the problem of TB screening by finding the right places and reaching out to those people most at risk is not sufficient – neither for disease control nor for the treatment of those unfortunate enough to have the disease. Active screening of the people empirically known to be at high risk is a politically pragmatic reaction to their vulnerability, yet it does not lead to a practical solution to cure them from a curable disease.

The screening measure I talked about played out in a socio-political context, where access to healthcare for the Roma is extremely difficult and where, additionally, French immigration policies have restricted their residential rights. The European polemic on the situation of the Roma in France in the summer of 2010 (Willsher 2010) is very relevant here, showing their extreme marginalisation in the public space (Nacu 2010). In her article 'Where ethics and politics meet', Miriam Ticktin (2006: 36) shows how a political 'climate of closure' that led to immigration restrictions led to the extension of humanitarian reasoning about immigrants who suffer from disease. In the case of PrO-S-TB, this is partly also the case. Public structures like the local TB control service had to rely on humanitarian structures to tackle the problem of TB control, which is by law the duty of public health authorities, yet their intervention was in vain. Even if the purpose of the local screening policy is to include and treat through early diagnosis those people whose social exclusion puts them at great risk of active TB and diagnostic delay, exclusionary immigration policies interfered, creating adverse conditions of care. The consequence is a paradoxical medical situation: abstaining from treating the most vulnerable patients despite successful diagnostic screening and readily available medication for a treatable disease.

Conclusion

What I described in the last section is an ethically tragic situation where it became politically impossible to treat those discovered through active screening to be most at risk for TB. The last example, as well as others, lead me to conclude that on a practical public health level, the active screening of migrants for TB needs to be reconceptualised. This could be done via the production of politically more meaningful epidemiological data, by supporting local knowledge, creativity and reflexivity, and by more closely articulating the nexus of TB screening and care. I have argued that migrants as an at-risk group are conceptualised in France and Germany in bureaucratic epidemiological disease surveillance data through crude categories such as nationality or place of birth. These categories do not sufficiently take into account the migrants' heterogeneous risk profiles in the country of immigration, which are very much influenced by their social situation and legal status, in short, their 'condition as migrant patient' (Fassin 2001), which differs greatly from one national context to another and between different migrant groups. Routine national epidemiological surveys, which should inform TB control policies, thus lack precise and localised data for those people most in need of screening and care. A first step to remedy this situation would be to include more information in the mandatory declarations, such as the legal status of migrants and their social security status, as well as data on the diagnostic context as has been implemented in France since 2010.

I have further argued that the public health objectives of targeted screening, namely, to treat those most vulnerable to TB, need to be articulated with the actual and often adverse political conditions of care, which are very dissimilar as they address differentially marginalised groups in different countries. If this is not done, even the most efficient targeted screening programme remains a symptomatic gesture towards controlling disease rather than a realistic option for treating people. My study thus shows the inherently political character of TB screening, particularly when Roma patients are concerned. Roma patients are paradoxical medico-political subjects, as their medical treatment interferes with different 'legal-administrative referentials' (Fassin 2001: 141). They are approached through two types of public politics that are mutually exclusive: an inclusionary one in the case of local disease control, and an exclusionary one in the case of national border control. In the current political climate it is the exclusionary approach that determines their conditions of care. Yet this does not go without contestation from health professionals. The screening and treatment of migrants are not only an example of caregivers' struggle with social inequalities and national policies, which play out differently according to the 'migrants' condition' (Fassin 2001: 139); they are also political practices, which are implemented on contested terrains.

Finally, using the example of a screening activity targeting particularly vulnerable migrants, my study shows that it is not stigmatising and surveilling public health measures that are most dangerous for migrants, as social science studies investigating migrant screening have held so far, but their ineffectiveness, given political closure and social inequalities. My study has thus raised pragmatic political issues that have not been studied sufficiently by sociologists and anthropologists in regard to screening and at-risk groups so far. Yet such studies seem important for future research and might help to add to studies on the surveillance and control of at-risk groups, which are mainly based on discourse analyses and tend not to engage sufficiently with the practical and political problems that are of primary importance: the definition and operationalisation of group risk, access to diagnostic screening and the nexus of screening and care. From my ethnographic study I found that it is these topics that need to be integrated in the sociology of screening, especially when vulnerable migrants are concerned. On a theoretical level, problems of in/visibility and inclusion/exclusion that are the corollary effects of social segregation and discrimination (Farmer 2003, Fassin 2000) would need to be treated more closely, as well as the practical problems of treatment after diagnostic screening in medically clear, yet politically adverse conditions of care.

Acknowledgements

I am very grateful to the public health professionals who shared their working and thoughts with me. My gratitude also goes to Manuel Schwab, Natalie Armstrong, Helen Eborall and the anonymous reviewers of the *Sociology of Health & Illness* for their valuable and insightful comments on earlier versions of the manuscript. Thanks to Najla Rettberg for the English language editing. I warmly thank Didier Fassin and Stefan Beck, my PhD supervisors, for many stimulating discussions, as well as my graduate institutions for logistic support: the Institut de recherche interdisciplinaire sur les enjeux sociaux at the Ecole des hautes études en sciences sociales Paris and the Institut für Europäische Ethnologie at Humboldt-Universität zu Berlin. The research was supported through a NaFöG PhD grant of the city of Berlin and a six-month fieldwork grant of the Centre interdisciplinaire d'études et de recherches sur l'Allemagne.

Notes

1   In some European countries, as is the case for France and other former colonial powers (Welshman and Bashford 2006), immigrants were targeted for TB screening early on. In France foreign workers have been screened on entering the country since the late 1940s (Wluczka 2007). For the past few years, at-entry screening for migrants has come under severe criticism and demands for its revision are made on account of its doubtful efficacy – economically as well as in regard to public health outcomes (Coker 2006, Dasgupta and Menzies 2005, Hargreaves *et al.* 2009, Klinkenberg *et al.* 2009).
2   For this argument, see also Kehr (2011) on TB contact-tracing and the thickness of social lives.
3   As TB is a notifiable disease, mandatory declarations are the primary source of national TB statistics. They are produced by French and German public disease surveillance institutions: the Institut de veille sanitaire in France and the Robert Koch-Institute in Germany.
4   The name is a pseudonym.

References

Antoine, D. (2006) *Tuberculose et migrations internationales en Europe de l'Ouest.* Nanterre: Université Paris X Nanterre.
Antoine, D. and Che, D. (2010) Epidemiologie de la tuberculose en France: bilan des cas déclarés en 2008, *Bulletin epidé miologique hebdomadaire,* 27–28, 6, 289–93.

Arshad, S., Bavan, L., Gajari, K., Paget, S.N.J., *et al.* (2010) Active screening at entry for tuberculosis among new immigrants: a systematic review and meta-analysis, *European Respiratory Journal*, 35, 6, 1336–45.

Barnes, D. (1995) *The Making of a Social Disease: Tuberculosis in Nineteenth-Century France*. Berkeley: University of California Press.

Bashford, A. (2010) The Great White Plague turns alien: tuberculosis and immigration in Australia, 1901–2001. In Condrau, F. and Worboys, M. (eds) *Tuberculosis Then and Now. Perspectives on the History of an Infectious Disease*. Montreal and Kingston: McGill-Queen's University Press.

Borde, T. and David, M. (2003) *Gut versorgt? Migrantinnen und Migranten im Gesundheits- und Sozialwesen*. Frankfurt am Main: Mabuse Verlag.

Bouchaud, O. (2009) Health care of vulnerable populations infected with TB and HIV, *Bulletin epidémiologique hebdomadaire*, 12–13, 119–21.

Brodhun, B., Altmann, D. and Haas, W. (2007) *Bericht zur Epidemiologie der Tuberkulose in Deutschland für 2005*. Berlin: Robert Koch-Institut.

Broekmans, J.F., Migliori, G.B., Rieder, H.L., Lees, J., *et al.* (2002) European framework for tuberculosis control and elimination in countries with a low incidence: recommendations of the World Health Organization (WHO), International Union Against Tuberculosis and Lung Disease (IUATLD) and Royal Netherlands Tuberculosis Association (KNCV) Working Group, *European Respiratory Journal*, 19, 4, 765–75.

Brown, T. (2000) AIDS, risk and social governance, *Social Science & Medicine*, 50, 9, 1273–84.

Carde, E., Fassin, D. and Ferré, N. (2002) Un traitement inégal. Les discriminations dans l'accès aux soins, *Migrations études*, 106, 1–10.

Coker, R. (2004) Compulsory screening of immigrants for tuberculosis and HIV, *British Medical Journal*, 328, 7435, 298–300.

Coker, R. (2006) Tuberculosis screening in migrants in selected European countries shows wide disparities, *European Respiratory Journal*, 27, 4, 801–7.

Comité national d'élaboration du programme de lutte contre la tuberculose (2007) *Programme de lutte contre la tuberculose en France 2007–2009*. Paris.

Craig, G.M. (2007) 'Nation', 'migration' and 'tuberculosis', *Social Theory and Health*, 5, 267–84.

Dasgupta, K. and Menzies, D. (2005) Cost-effectiveness of tuberculosis control strategies among immigrants and refugees, *European Respiratory Journal*, 25, 6, 1107–16.

David, M. (2001) *Migration und Gesundheit: Zustandsbeschreibung und Zukunftsmodelle*. Frankfurt am Main: Mabuse Verlag.

Desrosieres, A. (2000) *La politique des grands nombres. Histoire de la raison statistique*. Paris: La Découverte.

Diel, R. (2007) Prävention und Kontrolle der Tuberkulose, *Der Pneumologe*, 4, 3, 187–93.

Diel, R., Rusch-Gerdes, S. and Niemann, S. (2004) Molecular epidemiology of tuberculosis among immigrants in Hamburg, Germany, *Journal of Clinical Microbiology*, 42, 7, 2952–60.

Dubos, R. and Dubos, J. (1987) *The White Plague: Tuberculosis, Man, and Society*. New Jersey: Rutgers University Press.

Farmer, P. (2003) *Pathologies of Power. Health, Human Rights, and the New War on the Poor*. Berkeley, Los Angeles and London: University of California Press.

Fassin, D. (2000) Repenser les enjeux de santé autour de l'immigration, *Homme et Migration*, 1225, 5–12.

Fassin, D. (2001) Une double peine. La condition sociale des immigrés malades du sida, *L'Homme*, 160, 137–62.

Fearnley, L. (2010) Epidemic intelligence. Langmuir and the birth of disease surveillance, *Behemoth: A Journal on Civilisation*, 3, 3, 36–56.

Ferlinz, R. (1996) Die Tuberkulose in Deutschland und das Deutsche Zentralkommitee zur Bekämpfung der Tuberkulose, In Konietzko, N. (ed.) *100 Jahre Deutsches Zentralkommitee zur Bekämpfung der Tuberkulose (DZK). Der Kampf gegen die Tuberkulose*. Frankfurt am Main: PMI Verlagsgruppe.

Glaser, B.G. and Strauss, A.L. (1967) *The Discovery of Grounded Theory: Strategies for Qualitative Research*. Chicago: Aldine Publishing Company.

Hargreaves, S., Carballo, M. and Friedland, J. (2009) Screening migrants for tuberculosis: where next? *Lancet Infectious Disease*, 9, 3, 139–40.

Hauer, B., Kunitz, F., Sagebiehl, D., *et al.* (2006) *Abschlussbericht. Untersuchungen zur Tuberkulose in Deutschland: Molekulare Epidemiologie, Resistenzsituation und Behandlung*. Berlin: Deutsches Zentralkommitee zur Bekämpfung der Tuberkulose.

Huschke, S. (2011) Die Grenzen humanitärer Versorgung. In Bornschlegel, W., Frewer, A. and Mylius, M. (eds) *Medizin für Menschen ohne Papiere: Menschenrechte und Ethik in der Praxis des Gesundheitssystems*. Göttingen: VandR unipress.

Ho, M. (2004) Sociocultural aspects of tuberculosis: a literature review and a case study of immigrant tuberculosis, *Social Science & Medicine*, 59, 4, 753–62.

Keane, V. and Gushulak, B. (2001) The medical assessment of migrants: current limitations and future potential, *International Migration*, 39, 2, 29–42.

Kehr, J. (2009) The politics and poetics of migrant tuberculosis: modelling a 'social disease' in French public health. In Kalitzkus, V. and Twohig, P.L. (eds) *The Tapestry of Health, Illness and Disease*. Amsterdam: Rodopi.

Kehr, J. (2010) Geographien der Gefahr. Warum wieder über die Tuberkulose gesprochen wird. In Dilger, H. and Hadolt, B. (eds) *Medizin im Kontext. Krankheit und Gesundheit in einer vernetzten Welt*. Frankfurt am Main: Peter Lang Verlag.

Kehr, J. (2011) L'épaisseur des vies sociales. A propos du dépistage de la tuberculose. In Vailly, J., Kehr, J. and Niewöhner, J. (eds) *De la vie biologique à la vie sociale. Approches sociologiques et anthropologiques*. Paris: La Découverte.

King, N.B. (2003) Immigration, race and geographies of difference in the tuberculosis pandemic. In Gandy, M. and Zumla, A. (eds) *The Return of the White Plague: Global Poverty and the New Tuberculosis*. London: Verso Press.

Krieger, N. (2001) Theories for social epidemiology in the 21st century: an ecosocial perspective, *International Journal of Epidemiology*, 30, 4, 668–77.

Lang, T., Kelly-Irving, M. and Delpierre, C. (2009) Inégalités sociales de santé: du modèle épidémiologique à l'intervention. Enchaînements et accumulations au cours de la vie, *Revue d'Épidémiologie et de Santé Publique*, 57, 6, 429–35.

Lupton, D. (1999) *Risk and Sociocultural Theory. New Directions and Perspectives*. Cambridge: Cambridge University Press.

Marcus, G.E. (1995) Ethnography in/of the world-system. The emergence of multi-sited ethnography, *Annual Review of Anthropology*, 24, 95–117.

Mbaye, E.M. (2009) La santé des immigrés en France: controverses autour d'un paradigme, *Hommes et Migrations*, 1282, 6–19.

Mol, A. (2001) *The Body Multiple: Ontology in Medical Practice*. Durham: Duke University Press.

Nacu, A. (2010) Les Roms migrants en région parisienne: les dispositifs d'une marginalisation, *Revue européenne des migrations internationales*, 26, 1, 141–60.

Nader, L. (1994) Comparative consciousness. In Borofsky, R. (ed.) *Assessing Cultural Anthropology*. New York: McGraw-Hill.

Petersen, A. and Lupton, D. (1996) *The New Public Health: Health and Self in the Age of Risk*. London: Sage.

Pope, C. (2005) Conducting ethnography in medical settings, *Medical Education*, 39, 12, 1180–7.

Rieder, H.L., Zellweger, J.P., Raviglione, M.C., Keizer, S.T., *et al.* (1994) Tuberculosis control in Europe and international migration, *European Respiratory Journal*, 7, 8, 1545–53.

Savage, J. (2000) Ethnography and health care, *British Medical Journal*, 321, 7273, 1400–2.

Ticktin, M. (2006) Where ethics and politics meet, *American Ethnologist*, 33, 1, 33–49.

Veen, J., Migliori, G.B., Raviglione, M.C., *et al.* (2011) Harmonisation of TB control in the WHO European region: the history of the Wolfheze Workshops, *European Respiratory Journal*, 37, 4, 950–9.

Welshman, J. and Bashford, A. (2006) Health screening. Tuberculosis, migration, and medical examination: lessons from history, *Journal of Epidemiology and Community Health*, 60, 4, 282–4.

Welshman, J. (2000) Tuberculosis and ethnicity in England and Wales, 1950–1970, *Sociology of Health & Illness*, 22, 6, 858–82.

Welshman, J. (2010) Importation, deprivation, and susceptibility. Tuberculosis narratives in postwar Britain. In Condrau, F. and Worboys, M. (eds) *Tuberculosis Then and Now. Perspectives on the History of an Infectious Disease*. Montreal: McGill-Queen's University Press.

Willsher, K. (2010) France's deportation of Roma shown to be illegal in leaked memo, say critics, *The Guardian*. Available at http://www.guardian.co.uk/world/2010/sep/13/france-deportation-roma-illegal-memo (last accessed 15 September 2011).

Wluczka, M. (2007) Du contrôle sanitaire à la prévention, les enjeux de la santé des migrants, *Les Tribunes de la santé*, 17, 4, 39–45.

8

'Let's have it tested first': choice and circumstances in decision-making following positive antenatal screening in Hong Kong

Alison Pilnick and Olga Zayts

Introduction

As Reid *et al.* (2009) note, there has been a proliferation of qualitative sociological research examining antenatal screening for fetal chromosomal abnormalities since the late 1990s. Pilnick (2004, 2008) has suggested that this focus may in part be explained by two reasons. Firstly, the spectre of eugenics hangs heavy over fields of medical practice associated with genetics; and secondly, since termination of pregnancy is generally the only medical 'intervention' that can be provided if anomalies are confirmed, profound social and ethical issues are raised by the process. As a result, there have been a range of sociological studies examining women's decision-making regarding screening, often with a focus on choices and how these are experienced (e.g. Green and Statham 1996, Heyman *et al.* 2006, Markens *et al.* 1999, Markens *et al.* 2009, Reid *et al.* 2009, Reminnick 2006, Rothman 1988, Williams *et al.* 2005). A common theme emerging from this work is that women report that they have not felt able to exercise choice freely, experiencing constraints from both medical professionals and their perceived expectations of the sociocultures in which they live. As a result, women report accepting screening 'in order that this goes right', or because they see a failure to do so as 'unfair' to the baby (Press and Browner 1997).

While these sociological studies undoubtedly provide useful insights into women's decision-making, they mostly fail to reflect on the *actual* processes through which decisions are negotiated. They also run the risk that participants' reports of process are coloured by eventual outcomes of screening. Conversation analytic studies in other medical contexts have demonstrated the benefits of a close examination of how decisions are negotiated in real time through talk. These studies have shown various forms that patients' contributions to decision-making may take and the ways in which these contributions may be constrained by 'medical authority' (Collins *et al.* 2005: 2622); that is the medical contexts where these interactions take place and the contributions by the medical professionals (e.g. Stivers 2002, 2005, Koenig 2011, Toerien *et al.* 2011).

The Sociology of Medical Screening, First Edition. Edited by Natalie Armstrong and Helen Eborall. Chapters © 2012 The Authors. Book Compilation © 2012 Foundation for the Sociology of Health & Illness / Blackwell Publishing Ltd. Published 2012 by Blackwell Publishing Ltd.

This study builds on the foundations laid by the previous sociological and conversation analytic studies and pursues three interrelated objectives. Firstly, by employing conversation analysis it aims to examine the actual decision-making process in the specific context of antenatal screening. Secondly, the study looks at the 'next' stage in the process of antenatal screening, by focusing exclusively on women who have received 'positive' (high-risk) results from the initial screening process, and are subsequently being offered amniocentesis, an invasive diagnostic test which poses a risk of miscarriage of 0.5 to 1% (Leung *et al.* 2004). Understandably, these women represent an under-researched group, for a number of reasons: the delicacy of their circumstances; the smaller numbers involved; and the attendant ethical and practical difficulties in recruiting them. Whilst this group have been researched (e.g. Chiang *et al.* 2006, Markens *et al.* 2009), this research has been largely interview based, and sometimes aimed at evaluating specific outcomes of the consultations such as women's understanding of the screening results (Quagliarini *et al.* 1998, Statham and Green 1993) or their level of distress and its impact on decision-making (Marteau 1993, Weinans *et al.* 2000). Thirdly, the study site in Hong Kong provides a particularly interesting location in which to examine the process of antenatal screening, given limited available research in that part of the world and the diversity of client population receiving antenatal services due to the cosmopolitan nature of the setting. This diversity of the client population provides a rich environment for pursuing the third objective of the study: to examine how clients' social and economic circumstances are brought into the decision-making process by both medical professionals and clients, and how this might impact on clients' choices regarding antenatal screening.

(Non)directiveness, neutrality and social circumstance

To explore the ways in which wider social issues, and in particular the women's socioeconomic circumstances, are brought into the decision-making process, we draw on both conversation analytic work examining neutrality and how aspects of patients' lifestyles are introduced and sustained in consultations, and wider medical sociological literature which examines how doctors actively interpret social characteristics of patients.

Traditionally, genetic counselling and antenatal screening have been governed by the principle of non-directiveness. It is widely understood to mean that the role of the person offering testing should be that of information provider, rather than decision maker, and that information should be presented in a neutral, non-judgmental manner (Kessler 1997, Weil *et al.* 2006). However, there has been considerable debate in both the medical and sociological literature about whether absolute non-directiveness is professionally desirable or interactionally achievable (Anderson 1999, Bosk 1992, Clarke 1991, Gervais 1993, Pilnick 2002, Shiloh 1996), since it potentially requires both complete suspension of expert professional judgment and an orientation to what may be *heard* as directive even if it is not produced or intended as such. Taking these subtleties into consideration means that directiveness may often be an unintended consequence of the interactional process of antenatal screening. Previous research has shown, for example, that screening may be offered in a context of 'presumed acceptance', so that unless the pregnant woman explicitly states that she does not wish to undergo it, it is assumed that it will take place (Pilnick 2008). Maynard (1986) has described how utterances that are accountably non-directive or neutral can still be 'collaboration implicative' via the use of various subtle interactional resources. However, the issue of how external factors might impact on the presence of directiveness and the extent to which these influence an interaction have been little explored.

Sociological research in other medical settings has demonstrated that patients' social circumstances may constitute one such influencing factor. In particular, it has shown how different patients presenting with identical symptoms may be treated differently by doctors as a result of assumptions that are made related to social characteristics of patients that doctors deem relevant to medical treatment (Sudnow 1969, Lutfey and McKinlay 2009). Influential work in medical sociology has also explored the differences between doctors' interactions with privately paying and publicly funded patients, concluding that in private medicine doctors are more likely to personalise their communication and be prepared to have their recommendations questioned, whereas in state funded care doctors offer a more impersonal product, and appeal to the authority of the institution in underscoring professional dominance (Strong [1979]2001, Silverman 1987). Related to this, Strong ([1979]2001) argued that doctors' interaction could be influenced by the degree of similarity or difference between doctor and patient, with those patients in professional occupations who were able to afford private healthcare being more likely to be regarded as similar and their 'good character' assumed. Where there was a high degree of difference, patients in social circumstances that were seen to be less desirable (lone motherhood, welfare recipiency etc) could gain greater alignment with doctors by *demonstrating* their good character in consultations, for example by explicitly asking the doctor for advice. However, little is known about the actual interactional processes on which these findings are based. Strong's work is largely based on verbatim note taking, which means that some details of the interaction are necessarily lost, and whilst Silverman's data were mostly audio-recorded, he rejected the comprehensive transcription needed for a detailed interactional analysis as too time-consuming (Silverman 1987: 7–8). In terms of more recent work, Lutfey and McKinlay's (2009) work is based on vignettes shown to doctors, and they suggest that future work should examine real consultations. Similarly, Sorjonen and colleagues' (2006) conversation analytic work on consultations in primary care highlights that existing research does not explain how and why what they call 'lifestyle' topics come to be introduced into consultations and whether they are sustained or not. Whilst their focus is on issues of eating, smoking, drinking and exercising, they nevertheless raise questions about how medical stances towards these factors are formulated. It is these interactional subtleties that we explore in this essay.

Data and methods

This research is part of a large interactional study of antenatal screening in Hong Kong, on- going since 2006, which involves a close collaboration between the research team at the Universities of Hong Kong and Nottingham and a Prenatal Diagnostics and Counseling Department of one public hospital.

In Hong Kong patients have a choice between private and public health sectors, and there is no catchment area for public hospitals. 80% of Hong Kong residents have been reported to prefer private sector to public (Improving Hong Kong's Healthcare System 2009). However, the hospital where the data were collected is unusual in the sense that it is a teaching/training hospital for a medical faculty of one of the universities in Hong Kong and boasts extensive facilities and a substantial number of professorial staff. In addition, the University also contributes to subsidising the services. Therefore, similar to other public hospitals, it attracts patients with low monthly incomes and with chronic illnesses that require frequent medical visits. However, due to its high reputation and facilities, the hospital is also popular among high income families.

Similar to other public hospitals[1], in the hospital where the data were collected antenatal screening is provided as part of routine antenatal services. The screening is organised as a multi-stage activity. First, women are introduced to it through information leaflets and a 15 minute video outlining the nature of Down's syndrome, available screening and diagnostic tests, and some psychosocial aspects of screening. This introduction is followed by a face-to-face meeting with a hospital nurse or a doctor in which the information from the leaflets and the video and the woman's personal risks are discussed. Those women who receive a 'high-risk' or 'positive' screening report are invited for a second consultation, in which the need for a decision about amniocentesis is discussed. If a client chooses amniocentesis, a third consultation is scheduled if Down's syndrome is diagnosed to explain the diagnosis and to discuss subsequent management.

In this essay our focus is on a particular group of women who have undergone initial antenatal screening procedures and have received high-risk results (in this setting a result of greater than 1 in 250 for the combined test, and greater than 1 in 320 for the integrated test which assesses additional screening markers[2]). During the writing of this essay, the screening programme underwent a reform: previously only women ≥35 years old at delivery were offered any form of antenatal screening or testing, with the option of initial screening (nuchal translucency and maternal blood tests) or proceeding directly to diagnostic (CVS or amniocentesis) tests; from July 2010 *all* pregnant women have been offered screening tests with diagnostic testing only offered to women who have received high risk results from the initial screening. While this change has several potential implications (for example, identifying a larger number of cases of fetal abnormalities, including in younger women; potentially reducing the risk of miscarriage by reducing uptake of invasive tests as a first choice option), it did not affect the recruitment rate for this project as the recruitment criteria had been set at women ≥35 years old at delivery.

According to the hospital statistics, in 2007–2009, 2062 women received antenatal screening services. Among those women, 299 (11.5%) received high risk results. The high number of high risk patients may be attributed to a higher risk among women ≥35 years in comparison to younger women (Tang *et al.* 1991) (statistics for the period after screening was introduced for women of all ages are not yet available). Of these women, 145 (49%) opted for amniocentesis and the rest declined further testing. Medical providers at the hospital anecdotally attribute this high declination rate in part to the fact that a significant proportion of these women are migrant workers who leave Hong Kong during their pregnancy.

The data set used in this essay consists of 14 consultations with an overall recording time of more than three hours. Following the standard Ethics Committee approval obtained from the University of Hong Kong and a Hospital Authority cluster overseeing the hospital where the data were collected, recruitment procedure involved a study nurse approaching potential participants and introducing the research project to them, before seeking consent to participate. The background of the recruited participants reflects the diversity of patient population at the hospital. They originate from various parts of Asia (Hong Kong, Mainland China, Philippines, Thailand and Indonesia), North and South America, Europe, New Zealand and Australia. Their socioeconomic background ranges widely from women employed as domestic workers to those in professional occupations. The age of the participants is from 35 to 41 years old.

The consultations we recorded are conducted by four medical providers (three doctors and one nurse), all of whom are Hong Kong Chinese. In the extracts that we have selected for this essay, two doctors participate (who are referred to as D1 and D2 in the transcripts). The time allocated for each consultation is 15 minutes, since the personnel who provide antenatal screening services in the hospital are also involved in provision of other antenatal services. In the consultations either English or Cantonese are used as the first or the second language of the participants. The consultations conducted in Cantonese were initially transcribed and then translated into English. Aware of the social, cultural and political challenges involved in any act of transcribing, and particularly so in transcribing translated data (Bucholtz 2007), we have paid particular attention to 'validating' (Peräkylä 2004) the translations of the transcripts. More specifically, the initial transcriptions and translations were done by two bilingual research assistants. Both the transcripts and their translation were verified by a bilingual member of the research team. As Peräkylä suggests, we have paid particular attention to 'the next speaker's interpretation of the preceding action' in our analysis (2004: 216). The analysis was conducted using conversation analytic techniques (Jefferson, as published in Atkinson and Heritage 1984, ten Have 2007).

Findings

In our analysis we argue that the widely varied social circumstances of those residing in Hong Kong have visible impacts on which decisions come ultimately to be accepted or seen as 'right'. In order to provide some context for this analysis, we begin by highlighting a phenomenon that recurs throughout the data: that doctors appear in some instances to be quite directive in these consultations, both explicitly by appearing to assume that testing will take place, and implicitly through the information which they offer or withhold in particular circumstances. Extract 1 demonstrates both these aspects; here the doctor is apparently reluctant to discuss Down's syndrome, or its implications, until after diagnostic testing has taken place. This is noteworthy because more information about Down's syndrome may be consequential to whether women proceed with diagnostic testing:

Extract 1
The participants in this consultation are the pregnant woman (P), her husband (H) and the doctor (D2). The woman is Hong Kong Chinese, and the consultation is conducted in Cantonese, the participants' native language. The woman is 37 years old and this is her first pregnancy. Both the patient and the husband are employed as clerical staff. She has received a risk factor of 1 in 244 from her screening test. The extract comes after the discussion of the patient's screening results and further testing options.

313	H:	If eh: unfortunately it's Down syndrome, (.) then what is going to
314		do next? (.)
315		(.)
316	D2:	Em:: we'll check if the baby has other congenital problems or not
317		(0.2) Down syndrome (.) children with Down syndrome .h do
318		you know their situation?
319		(0.2)
320	H:	I don't know. ((shakes his head and turns to P))
321	P:	°I know° =
322	H:	= You ↑know?
323	P:	Their faces, and- their faces are so obvious(.) .h and they have learning
324		disability =
325	D2:	= Yes.
326	P:	Mainly learning and intelligence disability
327	D2:	Yes.

328	P:	No other problems?
329		(0.2)
330	D2:	Um (.) Eh: Let's have it tested first.
331		(0.5)
332	P:	Huh huh huh huh huh [huh huh ((nasal laugh))
333	D2:	[because overall sometimes the risk
334		is low.
335		(0.5)
336	D2:	If the baby really has Down syndrome(.) it means that he (.) like
337		what your wife said (.) he has an extra chromosome(.) he
338		is slow in learning (.) from mildly to moderately mentally
339		handicapped (.) delay (0.2) But it doesn't mean that
340		you can't help the baby (.). ha

((11 lines are omitted where the doctor asks the patient how she knows about Down's syndrome, and the patient describes the voluntary work she has undertaken))

352	D2:	uh hmm (.) Right (.) righ, righ (.) So you know how they behave?
353		((P nods))
354	D2:	Ha. ((looking at S))
355		(..) ((H shows an unhappy face))
356	P:	If we got it (.) it means if the baby has Down's=
357	D2:	= Right.
358	P:	Then eh for the abortion, usually within how many weeks should
359		I do? =
360	D2:	= Before twenty four weeks.

In this extract, following discussion of testing, the doctor suggests that following a positive test for Down's syndrome they will also check for congenital problems (line 316). He then asks the couple if they know the 'situation' of children with Down's syndrome. Following a negative response from her partner, the pregnant woman produces a candidate answer (lines 323–326) which encompasses both physical and intellectual features which she then uses as a basis for seeking further information (Pomerantz 1988). However, when the patient seeks this further information by asking in line 328 if there are other problems, the doctor declines to answer, suggesting that this is an issue that can be addressed after the test results are received. In his work on antenatal screening for Down's syndrome, Heyman (2010) has noted how the complexity of the real world has to be simplified in presenting screening results, and that the construction of Down's syndrome as something with a countable frequency inevitably directs attention away from the variable nature of the condition. In this case however the woman is actively seeking such information, and her laughter in line 332 appears to express some resistance or unease when she fails to elicit it (Haakana, 2001). The doctor subsequently produces a rationale for delaying the discussion; 'because overall sometimes the risk is low', implying that this is not something which needs to be addressed yet as it may be hypothetical. Following some intervening talk about voluntary work the woman has undertaken with people with learning disabilities, the pregnant woman asks another question (lines 356–359), about the timing of a potential abortion. Interestingly, unlike the request for further information about Down's syndrome, this question is not deflected as something which does not need to be dealt with until a problem is confirmed, and the doctor gives an immediate and direct answer (line 360). Therefore, in this example, we argue that the doctor's directiveness is evidenced by declining to provide more information about Down's syndrome despite the woman explicitly seeking that information. The utterance 'Let's have it tested first' contains an assumption that testing should take place prior to this discussion, and framing future action in this way potentially has a significant impact on client decision-making. The examples to follow look at how similar influences on decision-making may occur in response to the external circumstances that are raised by women in the course of the consultations. Extract 2 is an example where such circumstances are apparent:

Extract 2
The participants in this consultation are the pregnant woman (P) and the doctor (D3). The woman is Filipina, and is employed as a domestic worker. The consultation is conducted in English, the participant's second language. This is the woman's second pregnancy and she has one child. She has received a risk factor of 1 in 200 from her screening test. The extract comes after the delivery of the screening result.

30	D1:	.h so um it's up to you (.) We- we- we still call it screen positive (.)
31		Because there is a small possibility that the baby may have Down's.
32		(0.2)
33	P:	Um hmm.
34	D1:	.hh Em but it's up to you whether you want the amniocentesis: (.) em:
35		to check if [the baby has Down's
36	P:	[is it the- the one that put inside?
37		(0.2)
38	D1:	Yes, yes. ((while nodding))
39	P:	Hhh ((nasal laugh)) I've discussed it with my husband(.)He said
40		he doesn't want (.) Heh heh =
41	D1:	= Right ((while nodding))
42	P:	Because I still need to°work°
43		(0.3)
44	D1:	You- you worry that might give you =
45	P:	= Mis[carriage.
46	D1:	[Miscarriage (.) Ok (.) so, it's up to you because the chance that
47		the baby have a ah really have Down's is quite low =
48	P:	= °Um.°
49	D1:	It's only less than one percent (.) ok?
50		(0.2)
51	P:	Ummm.
52	D1:	So if you don't want that test, it's fine (.) Ok?
53		(0.2)
54	P:	°I don't think so.°
55	D1:	Ok. ((while nodding))

It is notable that the doctor's talk which introduces the amniocentesis in this consultation has a tentative quality and there is no use of any formulation that would include the doctor as an agent in any action, in contrast with 'Let's get it tested first' in Extract 1. Instead, in lines 30 and 34 the doctor explicitly labels it as the patient's decision and does not press a particular viewpoint (using 'it's up to you' twice). One immediately evident reason for this might be the relatively low risk figure. Previous sociological work in other medical contexts has shown that diagnostic certainty is a significant predictor of clinical action (Lutfey and McKinlay 2009), so that in cases of perceived high certainty there is more likely to be a proposed action. On the face of it, the relatively low risk here might appear to explain the doctor's refraining from producing such a proposal. However, any straightforward link between risk factor and degree of directiveness in this context is undermined by the fact that there are instances of women in our data with lower risk (e.g. Extract 1) where it is apparently assumed that testing will take place. We would argue that the lack of directiveness in respect of undergoing amniocentesis here may be explained by other aspects of this consultation. Following the pregnant woman's request for clarification about the invasive nature of amniocentesis ('Is it the one that put inside?' in line 36), and a confirmation from the doctor, the woman initially produces a response which gives her husband's view that testing isn't wanted. The doctor acknowledges this, and the patient subsequently produces a rationale to support this, that she 'needs to work' (line 42). We have been unable to find any comparable published data which references the need to work as the primary rationale for refusing amniocentesis[3], but we note here that the doctor's response does not treat it as unusual or surprising in any way. Instead, the doctor's response begins to propose a candidate explanation linking the need to work with the refusal of testing; a fear that working, rather than resting, after an amniocentesis test might increase the risk of miscarriage. The pregnant woman completes this candidate explanation herself, confirming this implied link. The doctor's response to this (lines 46–47) contains an affiliative overlap (Goldberg 1990), forecasting the subsequent acceptance of the woman's decision, on grounds that since the risk is quite low, it is okay not to want the test. As a result, the woman subsequently successfully declines the test.

Of particular interest to us here, then, is the fact that the doctor appears to accept at face value the rationale for rejecting the amniocentesis, the 'need to work' which potentially raises the risk of miscarriage associated with the test. This is in direct contrast with what occurs in Extract 3 below:

Extract 3

The participants in this consultation are the pregnant woman (P), her husband (H), and the doctor (D3). This is the woman's fifth pregnancy, and she has three children. She is 36 years old, and she has received 1 in 170 risk factor from the screening test. The couple are a high-income expatriate family from the UK. The consultation is conducted in English. This extract comes after the discussion of the actual procedure involved in amniocentesis, and how soon or long after the test miscarriage might occur.

801	H:	Um: there's no real recovery, per se, you're- you're just normal
802		or [(°etc°)
803	D1:	[no, em: (.) I mean just avoid sort of heav:y em housework =
804	H:	= Yeh ok. [Ok yeh. Huh huh
805	P:	[hh <h °Yeh that's good.° h> [huh huh huh
806	D1:	[hah hah hah [and em
807	H:	[°XXXX°
808	D1:	vigorous exercise =
809	P:	= Yeh.
810	D1:	Today or tomor[row
811	H:	[ok (.) so (.) ok
812	D1:	You don't need to rest in bed =
813	P:	= Yeh (.) [I know
814	D1:	[And It doesn't he[lp. .hh Ok?
815	H:	[Sure. Sure
816		(0.3)
817	D1:	But in case you have bleeding or if you have leakage after the

818		procedure (.) then you would need to rest in bed
819		(0.2)
820	H:	Ri[ght
821	P:	[Ok

In this extract, following the information that is given about the amniocentesis procedure, the husband asks a question about the recovery (line 801). This question is negatively framed (Raymond 2003), in that it projects a 'no' answer, and the doctor concurs that there is no real recovery period, advising that the woman should 'just avoid sort of heav:y em housework'. The way this utterance is produced, with its stretch on 'heavy', implies that non-heavy housework is not necessarily problematic. Equally, the use of 'just' serves to imply that this is the only everyday activity that should be avoided, though vigorous exercise (line 808) is later added to this list. This ability to carry on more or less as normal is subsequently reinforced in line 812, with the doctor's utterance 'You don't need to rest in bed', which is subsequently upgraded to a suggestion that this is neither necessary nor desirable ('And it doesn't help' in line 814). This sequence is closed by the doctor further asserting that bleeding or leakage are the only reasons for bed rest following the procedure.

Whilst this extract is interesting in its own right, it is particularly interesting in comparison to Extract 2. In Extract 3 above, the doctor seems at pains to ensure that the patient does not rest unnecessarily. In Extract 2, however, the doctor does not pursue either the fact that amniocentesis would only have a minimal effect on the patient's ability to work, or later clarify any increased risk of miscarriage associated with this. Neither does she ascertain whether the reported view of her husband is shared by the woman herself. Additionally, the 'need to work' expressed by the woman in Extract 2 is not in itself contested. As Sorjonen et al. (2006: 356) note, when an overt orientation to a problem is displayed in a patient's initial answer, 'it strongly proposes that the doctor take up the problem orientation in his subsequent turn'. The fact that the doctor in Extract 2 appears to align with the 'problem' of work is, then, what might be expected from the interactional literature. However, this explanation fails to hold for other instances in our data. Extract 4 is another example of a consultation in which work, and the inflexibility of work, is introduced as a factor in decision-making, but where it is dealt with rather differently.

Extract 4
The participants in this consultation are the woman (P), her husband (H) and the doctor (D3). The couple are high income Hong Kong Chinese, and the consultation is conducted in Cantonese, the participants' native language. The woman is 35 years old, and this is her first pregnancy. From the screening report her risk is 1 in 27. This extract comes after the discussion of process of amniocentesis.

691	H:	After amniocentesis what will be the mother's
692		[reaction?
693	D1:	[the mother we usually ask her not to work on that day.(.)
694		we will give her a medical certificate for sick leave for one
695		day (.) she does not need to stay in bed (.) Because if she
696		does not do a lot of labour [it is okay.
697	H:	[because we will fly the day
698		after tomorrow.
699	D1:	Oh you will fly the day after tomorrow (.) where will you go to?
700	P:	To [Beijing.

701	H:	[Beijing.
702	D1:	Beijing (.) and for when will you come back? Very soon
703		[right]?
704	P:	[Wed]nesday
705	H:	[er] next Wednesday =
706	D1:	= Oh then you can consider having amniocentesis after you come back
707	H:	That means it is not suggested to do it [before we go?
708	D1:	[yes yes you have to
709		go(.)right? you have to fly (.) that is a lot of work [anyway it is labor=
710	P:	[hh.
711		((P sighs and looks at H))
712	D1:	[and you only have little time
713	H:	[yes so we =
714	D1:	= ok > if you [really if you really want < to do it = ((looks at P and H))
715	H:	[that is if we really want to do it.
716	D1:	= before you fly then you should do it today
717		(0.5)

As in Extract 3, this extract also begins with a question about the possible reaction to amniocentesis. In this case, in contrast to Extracts 2 and 3, the doctor offers the possibility of a medical certificate to provide exemption from work for a day, though once again emphasises that bed rest is not necessary. In lines 697–698 the husband raises a potential problem, that the couple are due to fly on a business trip to Beijing, which has been alluded to in passing earlier in the consultation without being oriented to as problematic. However, the doctor's 'Oh' marks the timescale as newsworthy, and implies a problematic stance towards this new information (Heritage 2002). This consultation is being conducted on a Thursday, so the fact that they are not due to return till the following Wednesday would potentially mean a week's delay to testing. Though at this point the couple have not explicitly stated that they would like testing, the undesirability of the delay is first expressed in the doctor's question 'very soon right?' in lines 702–703, which clearly has a preferred answer (Pomerantz, 1984). Initially the doctor suggests that testing can take place on their return, but following the husband's question about the inadvisability of having it beforehand, she subsequently in lines 708–709 asks whether the woman has to go on the business trip, asserting that flying is 'a lot of work'. However, the implied unchangeability of the arrangement, as a result of the woman's sigh, is allowed to stand, and in the final part of the consultation not shown here, testing is subsequently arranged for the same day. Here is another interesting contrast with Extract 2: in that case, the need of the woman to work is accepted at face value as an insurmountable obstacle. In this case, the need is firstly questioned, and then testing is arranged around this, so that it is not taken as an unresolvable barrier. One salient difference between the two consultations reproduced in Extracts 2 and 4 is in the risk factors that the two women have received: 1 in 200 as opposed to 1:27. While a higher risk factor may be one explanation for the doctor's readiness to make arrangements around the woman's circumstances for the test to be taken in Extract 4, it might be expected that the official recommendations around recovering from amniocentesis should apply to all women regardless of risk factor. Comparing the two extracts, in Extract 2 it is the pregnant woman who introduces the topic of 'necessary' work in relation to amniocentesis, and in Extract 4 it is the pregnant woman's husband. Together, they demonstrate that the introduction of external factors relating to work into both these consultations plays a significant role in how these interactions unfold, though with different outcomes. Since the same doctor conducts both consultations, one obvious explanation is that her assessments of the 'need to work' for these two women – and hence the differing constraints work imposes on them – appears to result in these quite different outcomes. Whilst the woman in Extract 2 is a low income Filipina domestic worker, the woman in Extract 4 is a high income Hong Kong Chinese business woman. The interaction with the former woman contains no suggestion from the doctor that time off work, or a short period of reduced duties, is or should be possible, and her 'need' to continue is taken as evident. The interaction with the latter woman both questions the need, and treats the woman as potentially having the ability and/or resources to override this need. Taken together, these consultations begin to show the complex ways in which counsellors can influence the acceptance or otherwise of invasive tests, and how this influence may potentially be based at least partly on actualities or assumptions relating to sociocultural circumstance.

The impact external factors (and the doctor's subsequent assessment of them) can have is also evident in Extract 5 below but in a rather different context. In this extract, the pregnant woman is Chinese from Mainland China, and the consultation is conducted in Cantonese, though this is not her native language. Based on the integrated screening test, she has been given a risk figure for Down's syndrome of 1 in 295.

Extract 5
The participants in this interaction are the pregnant woman (P) and the doctor (D2). The woman is 36 years old, and this is her second pregnancy. The extract comes after the doctor has described the amniocentesis procedure and goes on to suggest there are five things the woman needs to take into account when making her decision.

235	D2:	< h right h > (.) hh I think you mainly consider this one (.) Sometimes
236		the chance is (.) just a ↑bit higher =
237	P:	= °just a bit higher°
238	D2:	Then second, the <u>ultrasound</u> is normal .hh third, (.) you have to balance
239		(.) the risk of miscarriage caused by amniocentesis. .h Fourth, you have
240		to consider (.) hh em: (.) the baby, 240. I mean if
241	P:	°Umm°
242	D2:	if the baby has Down syndrome (.) are you <u>really</u> unable to take care of
243		him (.) something like that. .hh =
244	P:	= I think (.) I can't accept it (.) I can't take care of him Hhh
245		((nasal laugh)) ((looking at D and smiling in an embarrassed way))
246	D2:	E:: hmm, you have to consider how much you understand the
247		syndrome (.) Fifth (.) we can't guarantee that the baby is
248		hundred percent normal even if you have the amniocentesis
249		or ultrasound (.) We just test the things we have to know
250	P:	((nodding)) I see ((nodding)) =
251	D2:	= If the baby is born (.) we discover he has another problem (.)
252		we can't say if we can accept it or not, right? So (.) if you think
253		you can accept an abnormal baby (.) then take it
254		(0.2)
255	P:	I'm afraid that I really can't take care of the baby if he has any
256		problems. huh huh huh
257	D2:	°Do you? Are you looking after one child? °=
258	P:	= Yes. I am living with my son (.) I'm single
259	D2:	°I see°. How old is he?
260	P:	He's in primary three

261	D2:	°That means you have to look after two children alone? °=
262	P:	= Yes (.) I have to work (.) so my mum helps me with this
263		(0.3)
264	D2:	Okay (0.2) Perhaps you may discuss it with your mother =
265	P:	= Mmm
266		(0.2)
267	D2:	It's not that urgent to decide now (.) Do you have the number of
268	D2:	Ms. X ((clinic nurse))?

At the beginning of this extract, then, the doctor is quite equivocal about testing. In listing the five things the patient needs to think about, she highlights in first and second place that the risk is only slightly higher than what would be considered normal for the patient's age, and that the ultrasound showed no visible abnormality. Thirdly, she raises the need to consider the risk of miscarriage associated with testing. This construction (minimising risk of abnormality whilst highlighting possible risk of procedure) serves to create a context in which testing is not the favoured option, and this is continued with her production of 'if the baby has Down syndrome are you really unable to take care of him' in lines 242–243, where the emphasis on 'really' suggests a contrast between what might be ideal and what is practically possible. The subsequent pause potentially indicates an upcoming dispreferred response (Pomerantz 1984), and the woman responds by stating in line 244 that she could neither accept nor take care of a child with a disability, with the latter formulation echoing the doctor's 'really unable to take care of' in line 242. The impact of this utterance is somewhat mitigated by the use of 'I think', and the doctor does not immediately accept this statement as a rationale for testing, instead suggesting by her utterance in lines 246–247 ('you have to consider how much you understand the syndrome') that this response is not necessarily based on full information. This, then, is an oppositional turn in Vuchinich's (1986: 282) sense of the term, since it 'negates an utterance, action or self of a hearer'. She then adds a fifth point to her list of options to be considered – that no test can guarantee a 'normal' child. This utterance, following acknowledgement by the pregnant woman, is used to build an argument that not being able to 'accept' a child with a disability is an insufficient justification, since a child may be born with a disability not revealed by testing and at that point it is too late for a choice to be made. However, the pregnant woman resists the generalisation that 'no-one knows' and returns instead to the specifics of her own situation. She sustains her position (lines 255–256) reiterating that *she* specifically will be unable to care for the baby 'if he has any problems'. Her prefacing of this position with 'I'm afraid' indicates her recognition that this is likely to be seen as a dispreferred option in this context, but this reiteration can still be seen as counter-oppositional (Maynard 1985). Notable also is that the pregnant woman's responses in lines 244 and 255–256 are followed by laughter particles that, as Glenn (2003: 122) maintains, express the woman's resistance towards 'potentially problematic talk'. A subsequent exchange with the doctor reveals the patient's family circumstances – that she is single and already has one child, whom her mother helps her to care for. At this point, the doctor, who until then appears to have been strongly favouring the option of not testing, and who has twice failed to accept the woman's expressed inability to care for a disabled child as closing the sequence, suggests that the issue should be discussed with her mother (line 264). Writing on conflict termination, Vuchinich (1990) notes that compromise (when a concession offering is followed by acceptance of the offering) is one of several strategies for ending conflictual talk, and this is apparent here, in that the possibility of testing, previously not forthcoming, is now preserved. The woman's uptake is not markedly enthusiastic, but rather than continuing with the discussion or revisiting her previously implied request for amniocentesis, the doctor's final utterance in the sequence defers the decision-making to another time. Here, then, the doctor's view as expressed in the interaction appears to shift considerably, from an initial position, sustained over resistance from the pregnant woman, that testing is not necessary or desirable, to a position that testing is something that can be arranged following discussion with her mother, and by contacting the clinic nurse. Whilst the woman's own clearly expressed views have failed to bring about an offer of testing, the doctor's realisation that she is a single parent with another child appears to be the stimulus for preserving this possibility.

Discussion

We began this chapter by suggesting that Hong Kong is a particularly interesting setting in which to examine antenatal screening, given the diversity of its community. Previous work on antenatal screening has identified how women report feeling their choices are constrained by social and economic factors (Lam *et al.* 2000). We have focused our analysis particularly on consultations where these social and economic circumstances are interactionally visible, and the consequences that this presence has for how consultations unfold and how decisions are made and accepted or challenged. Women and their partners may raise work as a rationale for refusing testing, or being unable to undergo testing at the suggested or preferred time. They may also invoke other socioeconomic factors (e.g. being a lone parent) as a rationale *for* testing, on the basis that a child with Down's syndrome is not manageable for them. What is significant in these data is that once they have been raised, these issues are not necessarily treated in the same way, even by the same doctor. Only in some cases are these external factors, as presented by women or their partners, seen as unchangeable or insurmountable, so that 'a need to work', or 'an inability to cope' may be subject to further evaluation in the context of what is known about the women's social circumstances. In presenting our analysis, we have drawn on previous published work which has demonstrated how doctors actively interpret patients' social characteristics, and formulate stances towards lifestyle issues that patients raise (Sudnow 1967, Strong [1979]2001, Silverman 1987, Lutfey and McKinlay 2009, Sorjonen *et al.* 2006). What we have found here is considerably more subtle than the phenomena identified by Silverman and Strong; there is certainly no suggestion that interactions with patients from varying socioeconomic backgrounds are differently structured in any overarching sense. However, it does appear that when socioeconomic circumstances are made explicitly visible in consultations, the extent to which these are seen or allowed by doctors to impact on decision- making is subject to interpretation. Whilst we should not be surprised that such interpretation also occurs in the context of antenatal screening, the particular sensitivities of this area raise some specific issues. The linkage between lifestyle 'problems' in primary care, for example, (such as a high fat diet, or excessive alcohol consumption) are potentially much more straightforwardly mapped to outcomes (such as high cholesterol levels, or raised blood pressure). It can be argued that this mapping makes the taking of a stance by doctors less problematic, on grounds of medical justification. However, the way in which a woman or couple's social circumstances map on to the willingness or ability to care for a disabled child is far less easily imputable, and in the context of non-directive counselling there can be no recourse to medical justification.

Though this is a small sample and large scale generalisation is clearly not appropriate, differences in what are seen to be acceptable reasons for accepting or refusing testing do seem strongly linked to the different socioeconomic circumstances of these women and the assumptions that may be made as a result. These findings help us further understand the social and ethical implications of screening, and the way these implications are inextricably linked with the sociocultural contexts in which pregnant women live. They also add to the growing literature on the difficulty of achieving non-directiveness in antenatal screening, by highlighting some of the subtle and complex interactional processes through which counsellors may influence the acceptance or declination of invasive tests.

Acknowledgements

The research reported here was fully supported by a grant from the Hong Kong Research Grants Council of the Hong Kong Special Administrative Region, China (project no. HKU 754609 H). Thanks are due to all those involved with the project, particularly Alice Yau, and to the clinicians and pregnant women who allowed their consultations to be recorded.

Notes

1 Pregnant women also have a choice of undergoing antenatal screening in a private sector where the arrangements may differ depending on individual private doctors.
2 In Hong Kong non-invasive screening tests offered to pregnant women include an ultrasound measurement of nuchal thickness and maternal blood biochemical markers. These tests can be performed alone or in combination. The ultrasound measurement is performed at 11 to 14 weeks gestation, and it may be combined with maternal blood test (alpha-fetal protein, beta-hCG) at 16 to 19 weeks gestation. The detection rate for this combined test is around 80% at a screened positive rate of 5% (Lam *et al.* 2002). There is also an option of having an integrated test where a combined test is carried out at 11–14 weeks and another blood test is offered in the second trimester of pregnancy at 15–20 weeks. The integrated test has a higher detection rate and a lower false positive rate.
3 The lack of comparable incidents in published UK literature may be explained by the legal right in the UK to take time off to attend antenatal appointments.

References

Anderson, G. (1999) Nondirectiveness in prenatal genetics: patients read between the lines, *Nursing Ethics*, 6, 2, 126–36.
Atkinson, J.M. and Heritage, J. (eds) (1984) *Structures of Social Action: Studies in Conversation Analysis*. Cambridge: Cambridge University Press.
Bosk, C. (1992) *All God's Mistakes: Genetic Counselling in a Paediatric Clinic*. Chicago: University of Chicago Press.
Bucholtz, M. (2007) Variation in transcription. *Discourse Studies*, 9, 6, 784–808.
Cheng, W. (2003) *Intercultural Conversation*. Amsterdam: Benjamins.
Chiang, H.H., Chao, Y.M. and Yuh, Y.S. (2006) Informed choice of women in prenatal screening tests for Down's syndrome, *Journal of Medical Ethics*, 32, 273–7.
Clarke, A. (1991) Is non-directive genetic counselling possible? *Lancet*, 338, 959–1026.
Collins, S., Drew, P., Watt, I. and Entwistle, V. (2005). 'Unilateral' and 'bilateral' practitioner approaches in decision-making about treatment, *Social Science & Medicine*, 61: 2611–27.

Gervais, K.G. (1993) Objectivity, value neutrality, and nondirectiveness in genetic counseling. In Bartels, D.M., LeRoy, B. and Caplan, A.L. (eds) *Prescribing our Future: Ethical Challenges in Genetic Counseling*. New York: Aldine de Gruyter.

Glenn, P. (2003) *Laughter in Interaction*. Cambridge: Cambridge University Press.

Goldberg, J. (1990) Interrupting the discourse on interruptions, *Journal of Pragmatics*, 14, 883–903.

Green, J. and Statham, H. (1996) Psychosocial Aspects of Prenatal Screening and Diagnosis. In Marteau T. and Richards M. (eds) *The Troubled Helix: Social and Psychological Implications of the New Human Genetics*. Cambridge: Cambridge University Press.

Haakana, M. (2001) Laughter as a patient's resource: dealing with delicate aspects of medical interaction, *Text*, 21, 187–219.

Have, P. (2007) *Doing Conversation Analysis: A Practical Guide*. London: Sage.

Heritage, J. (2002) Oh-prefaced responses to assessments: A method of modifying agreement/ disagreement. In Ford, C.E., Fox, B.A. and Thompson, S. (eds) *The Language of Turn and Sequence*. Oxford: Oxford University Press.

Heyman, B. (2010) The social construction of health risks. In Heyman, B., Alaszewski, A., Shaw, M. and Titterton, M. (eds) *(2010) Risk, Safety and Clinical Practice: Health care through the lens of risk*. Oxford: Oxford University Press.

Heyman, B., Hundt, G., Sandall, J., Spencer, K., Williams, C., Grellier, R. and Pitson, L. (2006) On being at higher risk: A qualitative study of prenatal screening for chromosomal anomalies, *Social Science and Medicine*, 62, 2360–72.

Improving Hong Kong's Healthcare System: For Whom and Why? Report by the Harvard Team for the Health and Welfare Bureau of the Government of Hong Kong SAR. Retrieved on September 14, 2009 from http://www.fhb.gov.hk/en/press_and_publications/consultation/HCS.HTM.

Kessler, S. (1997) Psychological aspects of genetic counseling. XI: Nondirectiveness revisited. *American Journal of Medical Genetics*, 72, 164–71.

Koening, C.J. (2011) Patient resistance as agency in treatment decisions, *Social Science and Medicine*, 72, 7, 1105–14.

Lam, Y.H., Tang, H.Y., Lee, C.P., Sin, S.Y., Tang, R., Wong, H.S. and Wong, S.F. (2000) Acceptability of serum screening as an alternative to cytogenetic diagnosis of Down syndrome among women 35 years or older in Hong Kong, *Prenatal Diagnosis*, 20, 487–90.

Leung, T.N., Chau, M.M.C., Chang, J.J., Leung, T.Y., Fung, T.Y. and Lau, T.K. (2004) Attitudes towards termination of pregnancy among Hong Kong Chinese women attending prenatal diagnosis counselling clinic, *Prenatal Diagnosis*, 24, 546–51.

Lutfey, K. and McKinlay, J. (2009) What happens along the Diagnostic Pathways to CHD Treatment? Qualitative Results Concerning Cognitive Processes, *Sociology of Health and Illness*, 31, 7, 1077–92.

Markens, A., Browner, C.H. and Press, N. (1999) 'Because of the risks': How US pregnant women account for refusing prenatal screening, *Social Science and Medicine*, 49, 359–69.

Markens, S., Browner, C.H. and Preloran, H.M. (2009) Interrogating the dynamics between power, knowledge and pregnant bodies in amniocentesis decision making, *Sociology of Health and Illness*, 32, 1, 37–56.

Marteau, T.M. (1993) Psychological consequences of screening for Down's syndrome. Still being given too little attention, *British Medical Journal*, 307, 6897, 146–47.

Maynard, D. (1985) How children start arguments, *Language in Society*, 4, 1–20.

Maynard, D. (1986) Offering and soliciting collaboration in multiparty disputes among children (and other humans). *Human Studies*, 9, 261–85.

Peräkylä, A. (2004) Reliability and validity in research based on tapes and transcripts. In Silverman, D. (ed) *Qualitative Research: Theory, Method and Practice*. London: Sage.

Pilnick, A. (2002) 'There are no rights and wrongs in these situations': Identifying interactional difficulties in genetic counselling, *Sociology of Health and Ilness*, 30, 4, 511–30.

Pilnick, A. (2008) 'It's something for you both to think about': choice and decision making in nuchal translucency screening for Down's syndrome, *Sociology of Health and Illness*, 30, 4, 511–30.

Pilnick, A., Fraser, D. and James, D. (2004) Presenting and discussing nuchal translucency screening for fetal abnormality in the UK, *Midwifery*, 20, 1, 82–93.

Pomerantz, A. (1984) Agreeing and disagreeing with assessments: Some features of preferred/dispreferred turn shapes. In Atkinson, J.M. and Heritage, J. (eds) *(1984) Structures of Social Action: Studies in Conversation Analysis*. Cambridge: Cambridge University Press.

Pomerantz, A. (1988) Offering a candidate answer: An information seeking strategy, *Communication Monographs*, 55, 4, 360–73.

Press, N. and Browner, C.H. (1997) Why women say yes to prenatal diagnosis, *Social Science and Medicine*, 45, 979–89.

Quagliarini, D., Betti, S., Brambati, B. and Nicolini, U. (1998) Coping with serum screening for Down syndrome when the result is given as a numeric value, *Prenatal Diagnosis*, 18, 816–21.

Raymond, G. (2003) Grammar and social organization: yes/no interrogatives and the structure of responding, *American Sociological Review*, 68, 939–67.

Reid, B., Sinclair, M., Barr, O., Dobbs, F. and Crealey, G. (2009) A meta-synthesis of pregnant women's decision making processes with regard to antenatal screening for Down sydrome, *Social Science and Medicine*, 69, 1561–73.

Reminnick, L. (2006) The quest for the perfect baby: Why do Israeli women seek prenatal genetic testing? *Sociology*, 28, 1.

Rothman, B.K. (1988) *The Tentative Pregnancy: Prenatal Diagnosis and the Future of Motherhood*. London: Pandora.

Shiloh, S. (1996) Decision-making in the context of genetic risk. In Marteau, T. and Richards, M. (eds) *The Troubled Helix: Social and Psychological Implications of the New Human Genetics*. Cambridge: Cambridge University Press. pp. 82–103.

Silverman, D. (1987) *Communication and Medical Practice: Social Relations in the Clinic*. London: Sage.

Sorjonen, M-L., Raevaara, L., Haakana, M., Tammi, T. and Peräkylä, A. (2006) Lifestyle discussions in medical interviews. In Heritage, J. and Maynard, D. *(2006) Communication in Medical Care: Interaction between primary care physicians and patients*. Cambridge: Cambridge University Press.

Statham, H. and Green, J. (1993) Serum screening for Down's syndrome: Some women's experiences, *British Medical Journal*, 307, 174–6.

Stivers, T. (2002) Participating in decisions about treatment: overt parent pressure for antibiotic medication in pediatric encounters, *Social Science and Medicine*, 54, 1111–30.

Stivers, T. (2005) Parent resistance to physicians' treatment recommendations: one resource for initiating a negotiation of the treatment decision, *Health Communication*, 18, 41–74.

Strong, P. ([1979]2001) *The Ceremonial Order of the Clinic: Patients, doctors and medical bureacracies*. Aldershot: Ashgate.

Sudnow, D. (1967). *Passing on: The social organization of dying*. Englewood Cliffs, New Jersey: Prentice-Hall, Inc.

Tang, M., Ghosh, A. and Chan, F.Y. (1991) Genetic counselling in prenatal diagnosis, *Journal of the Hong Kong Medical Association*, 43, 2.

Toerien, M., Shaw, R., Duncan, R. and Reuber, M. (2011) Offering patients choices: A pilot study of interactions in the seizure clinic, *Epilepsy & Behavior*, 20, 312–20.

Vuchinich, S. (1986) On attenuation in verbal family conflict, *Social Psychology Quarterly*, 49, 4, 280–93.

Vuchinich, S. (1990) The sequential organization of closing in verbal family conflict. In Grimshaw, A.D. (ed) *Conflict Talk: Sociolinguistic investigations of arguments in conversations*. Cambridge: Cambridge University Press.

Weil, J., Ormond, K., Peters, J., Peters, K., Biesecker, B.B. and LeRoy, B. (2006) The relationship of nondirectiveness to genetic counseling: Report of a workshop at the 2003 NSGC Annual Education Conference, *Journal of Genetic Counseling*, 159, 2.

Weinans, M.J., Huijssoon, A.M., Tymstra, T., Gerrits, M.C., Beekhuis, J.R. and Mantingh, A. (2000) How women deal with the results of serum screening for Down syndrome in the second trimester of pregnancy, *Prenatal Diagnosis*, 20, 9, 705–8.

Williams, C., Sandall, J., Lewando-Hundt, G., Heyamn, B., Spencer, K. and Grellier, R. (2005) Women as moral pioneers? Experiences of first trimester antenatal screening, *Social Science and Medicine*, 6, 9, 1983–92.

9

Representing and intervening: 'doing' good care in first trimester prenatal knowledge production and decision-making

Nete Schwennesen and Lene Koch

Introduction

Current professional and policy debate over the use of prenatal testing emphasises the need for making informed choices and for services that provide prospective parents with what is referred to as 'non-directive counselling'. An increasing number of studies have focused on how current regimes of choice give rise to complex processes of decision-making for pregnant women and their partners, who are obliged to choose and thereby take full responsibility for serious decisions on life and death, on the basis of partial risk knowledge (Franklin and Roberts 2006, Rapp 2000, Rothman 1986, Schwennesen *et al.* 2010). Health professionals play an important role as facilitators of choice and as administrators of the official policy of autonomy and the knowledge, technologies and choices that are made available to the pregnant women and their partners. Nonetheless, only a few studies have focused on how regimes of choice are perceived, reflected on and acted upon by health professionals and how difficulties are experienced and handled in professional practice.

Studies focusing on professional practice of prenatal counselling tend to deal mainly with how professionals fail to live up to ideals of non-directiveness (Anderson 1999, Brunger and Lippman 1995, Hunt *et al.* 2005, Lippman 1991, Lupton 1999, Petersen 1999, Pilnick 2008, Williams *et al.* 2002). Empirical studies have demonstrated that while counsellors generally strive for non-directiveness in counselling, in everyday practice they frequently depart from it (Brunger and Lippman 1995, Williams *et al.* 2002). This gap between ideals and practices has been described as a serious problem of power, which eventually limits the possibilities of choice (Petersen 1999). Exploring some of the difficulties health practitioners encountered when attempting to work non-directively, Williams *et al.* (2002) found 'a variety of circumstances when nondirective counselling did not seem to be possible or to be the most appropriate response to the situation' (Williams *et al.* 2002: 345). These circumstances varied from 'acting in response to women's requests for directiveness, to covertly making decisions on behalf of women' (Williams *et al.* 2002: 345). On this basis Williams and colleagues suggest

The Sociology of Medical Screening, First Edition. Edited by Natalie Armstrong and Helen Eborall. Chapters © 2012 The Authors. Book Compilation © 2012 Foundation for the Sociology of Health & Illness / Blackwell Publishing Ltd. Published 2012 by Blackwell Publishing Ltd.

viewing prenatal counselling as a process that forms a continuum between choice and coercion and request 'discussions as to which – if any – aspects of directiveness are acceptable and which are not' (Williams *et al*. 2002: 345). In this article we wish to extend this discussion by relating it to the question of care. Whereas Williams *et al*. take as their starting point the ideal of non-directiveness for characterising, assessing and understanding professional practices, we take the clinical practices of care as a starting point for our analysis. In doing so, we are inspired by recent scholars in the field of science and technology studies (STS) who have taken up the question of care in relation to health practice (Despret 2004, Mol 2006, 2008, Mol *et al*. 2010, Pols 2003, Struhkamp *et al*. 2009). These scholars have been critical of the way in which abstract ideals such as autonomy and non-directiveness have come to colonise discussions on how to improve healthcare practices. We share this concern and seek to contribute to this move away from abstract ideals by articulating practices of care in the context of prenatal testing and counselling in Denmark, on the basis of ethnographic material.

The Danish case

New guidelines were issued by the Danish Board of Health in 2004 announcing a 'paradigm shift' from a paradigm of prevention towards one of self-determination (Danish Board of Health 2004). The Board wanted to signal a movement away from the previous practice of prenatal testing which, they argued, represented a prevention-oriented paradigm as it was organised around particular screening criteria such as age: only pregnant women of or above 35 years of age or women with a known increased risk of giving birth to a child with a chromosomal disorder were automatically eligible for prenatal testing. To counter what the Board considered a problematic prevention-oriented paradigm of the past, a new aim of future prenatal testing was introduced: the aim of informed choice. The main success criterion for the programme was therefore formulated as facilitating a space for action for the pregnant woman, where she would be able to make a decision in accordance with her own values and beliefs (Danish Board of Health 2004). Accordingly, it was emphasised that neutral information and non-directiveness in counselling was a precondition (Danish Board of Health 2004). This concurs with the general approval of the ideal of informed choice (Marteau *et al*. 2001) and the principle of non-directiveness in prenatal counselling[1] (Clarke 1997, Harper 2004, Harris *et al*. 1999, Hunt *et al*. 2005, Williams *et al*. 2002) and expresses a current tendency in European and American countries to frame choice and objective information as an obvious solution to what is considered a problematic prevention-oriented past of prenatal testing.[2]

The guidelines paved the way for introducing the technology of the first trimester prenatal risk assessment (FTPRA) offered to every pregnant woman in Denmark, regardless of age. The FTPRA is performed during the 11th to 13th gestational weeks and is a non-invasive method based on an ultrasound scan and maternal serum markers. It is considered one of the most effective non-invasive screening technologies for Down's syndrome and other chromosomal abnormalities (Nicolaides 2004, Williams et al. 2002) and has increasingly become a routine element of antenatal care in European countries (Pilnick 2008) and in the USA (Hunt *et al*. 2005). Denmark is a unique case: it is the first country in the world to introduce an FTPRA as a public health offer to every pregnant woman, regardless of age and risk situation and is free of charge.

Today, the FTPRA has become an almost routine part of pregnancy in Denmark. A recent study on the uptake of the FTPRA in Denmark shows that only 2% of couples offered an FTPRA during 1 July–31 December 2005 actively refused the offer. It is estimated that the overall current take-up is at least 90% which, to our knowledge, is one of the highest population uptakes worldwide (Tørring *et al.* 2008). In the Copenhagen area, where this study was conducted, take-up is estimated to be more than 95% (Tabor 2006, personal communication).

From non-directiveness to modes of doing good care

In the following we do not intend to evaluate whether the new ideals of non-directiveness and choice are actually realised in practice. Rather, we study the process through which knowledge and decisions are made in FTPRA trajectories. With inspiration from scholars in STS we adopt a constructivist ontology, which states that entities are not pre-existing practice but are entangled with each other in socio-material networks and gain their specific qualities through these relations (Latour 1987, Law 1994, Mol 2002). According to Rehmann-Sutter (2009) non-directiveness can be defined as providing completely unbiased information and a restraint from giving practical advice. From the perspective of STS, however, non-directiveness (understood as providing completely unbiased information) becomes absurd. Rather, attention is drawn to the acknowledgement that knowledge production is an intervention in itself with serious implications for those involved. As Foucault and Hacking have already taught us, knowledge may be conceived of as a powerful intervention, which brings forth new identities and relationships (Hacking 1986, Foucault 1978). If we take this point, the question of how to do good in health care practice can no longer meaningfully be thought of as how to avoid interference (non-directiveness) since knowledge production in itself – objective or not – must be conceived of as an intervention. Instead, attention is drawn to questions of interference, such as how to interfere with and be accountable for the new entities and phenomena that emerge through such knowledge production. If we apply this framework to the analysis of the FTPRA, we can think about it as an emergent process of knowledge production through which new forms of associations between humans and technology are made possible and new phenomena such as life and risk are made to matter. Who the pregnant woman is (mother/pregnant woman, responsible/irresponsible, empowered/victimised) and what the fetus becomes (human/non-human, low risk/high risk) might potentially change through the socio-material associations the pregnant woman engages with when she undergoes an FTPRA. This translation is symmetrical; the technologies involved in an FTPRA (the ultrasound scan, the risk assessment), what they are and what they do might also undergo a change.

In the following we identify modes of doing good care (Pols 2003) as they are played out in the process of knowledge production and decision-making in FTPRA trajectories. We define modes of 'doing' good care as a temporal way of ordering practice in entities (such as the human, the non-human, life, risk) which together form a pattern of relational meaning directed towards 'the good' (Boltanski and Thévenot 1991). We articulate such modes in relation to two obligatory points of passage (Latour 1987) that women and partners must go through during an FTPRA: (i) the performance of the ultrasound scan and (ii) the communication of a risk figure and the subsequent decision about what to do on this basis. We frame those points of passage as constitutive for the making and remaking of boundaries around life and risk and illustrate how such ordering practice happens through a temporal process of attunement (Despret 2004, Mol 2008) where hopes, expectations, technologies and humans are continuously made and modified in the clinical encounter.

The study

Over six weeks in 2005, the first author (NS) undertook observations of practice and had several informal conversations with sonographers at a Danish ultrasound clinic. During the observations of practice, NS focused particularly on problematic situations, how they occurred and how they were attempted to be handled in practice. In addition, six sonographers and one consultant (originally trained as a medical doctor) who teaches a certification course, were interviewed. The sonographers were presented with the problematic situations identified during participant observation and asked how they would attempt to handle such situations. They were also asked to define and give practical examples of problematic situations, explain why they saw those situations as particularly problematic and how they handled the situation in practice or how they would ideally handle the situation in practice. This method of articulating professional self-reflection is suggested by Mol (2006).

The sonographers were interviewed in their working hours and were chosen at random according to whichever sonographer was at work when the clinic schedule allowed time for an interview. The sonographers interviewed had between one and twenty years' working experience in the field and were aged 30 to 50 years. All of them were women and were living in Copenhagen or in the suburbs of Copenhagen. Two interviewees had originally trained as midwives and four as nurses; all were trained as sonographers according to the certification programme developed by the Fetal Medicine Foundation, based in the UK, emphasising correct measurement of ultrasound images, the statistics behind the risk calculation and the facilitation of informed choice through non-directive counselling.[3]

In relation to previous work, NS had also conducted 14 semi-structured interviews with pregnant women undergoing an FTPRA and their partners. This work has been published elsewhere (Schwennesen 2011, Schwennesen et al. 2009, 2010, Schwennesen and Koch 2009). Although these interviews are not analysed in this study, they framed our understanding of practice and are drawn on occasionally.

This study is not representative of professional practice of the FTPRA in Denmark or in general. The main contribution of this study is its attempt – through detailed empirical material – to illustrate the actual process through which knowledge is made in a particular institutional setting of the FTPRA and to articulate the different ways in which professionals seek to intervene in this process with care. Our hope is that such articulations may inform current debate on how to improve healthcare in prenatal testing and counselling.

There follows below an analysis of the two obligatory points of passage women and partners have to go through during an FTPRA: the scan, and the receipt of a risk figure and the subsequent decision. Within each point of passage we describe particular problematic situations as experienced by sonographers and articulate how such situations are handled with care.

The first point of passage: the ultrasound scan

Entering the scan; attuning knowledge and expectations
The pregnant woman[4] will be informed about the possibility of undergoing an FTPRA at the first pregnancy check-up with her general practitioner around week 8 of pregnancy. If she decides to attend an FTPRA she must book an appointment over the internet or by telephoning the hospital. Before attending the ultrasound scan, a serum test must be taken at the hospital between weeks 9 and 13. The ultrasound scan is undertaken between

weeks 11 to 13 of pregnancy and after the scan a final overall risk calculation is made and communicated to the pregnant woman. This provides the basis of whether an invasive test to obtain fetal material (amniocentesis or chorionic villus sampling) is offered. Such tests are diagnostic but involve the risk of inducing a miscarriage of a healthy child (around 1%) (Tabor *et al.* 1986).

In Denmark the FTPRA has become an almost obligatory point of passage for women on the trajectory towards giving birth. The entry into an FTPRA may therefore be described as a 'default pathway' (Webster 2007: 47) for pregnant women on the normal trajectory towards having a (healthy) baby, rather than an act of choice. This point is also made by a sonographer (S2): 'It is not something you choose, it is just something you do, it has become an act of routine'.

In interviews with NS the sonographers explained that they often experienced a problematic discrepancy between a woman's positive expectations when she enters the scanning room and their own professional understanding of the scan as a screening tool. One sonographer[5] says:

S1:   The attendees and the professional have two different approaches to the scan. We are trouble-shooters and perform the scan as part of a technology that aims to find something which is abnormal. At the same time many couples come with a positive attitude, where they expect everything to be fine and that they will have a look at their fetus for the first time.

The problematic situation referred to illustrates a gap between the woman's expectations of the scan as a technology of life confirmation and the underlying rationale of the FTPRA of identifying high-risk fetuses in order to prevent disease. The sonographers, however, enact the FTPRA as a screening technology to identify fetuses at risk with the aim of preventing disease. In cases where the resulting risk figure is interpreted as low risk, the pregnant woman's hope and expectations will be confirmed, as she will go home with a printed ultrasound picture, proving this to be the case. When the resulting risk figure is interpreted as high, however, the potentiality of a 'risky' future is brought into the present. In such cases the gap between the pregnant woman's expectations and how the risk assessment actually plays out, may show itself in feelings of shock, sadness and grief when she is confronted with the message of being classified as high risk.

To protect women from what the sonographers describe as 'unnecessary shock and nervousness', they explain how they attempt to reduce the gap by trying to reach a shared understanding of, and expectations about, what the FTPRA is before they start scanning. In doing so, the sonographers emphasise the importance of trying to get to know more about the particular pregnant woman by asking questions about background, family situation, previous experiences with the FTPRA and so on before they start scanning in order to adjust information and attune expectations. As one sonographer says:

S3:   They may be very nervous or they may have several other things going on in their lives, which take up a lot of space, such as a sick child, divorce or illness . . . they are positioned in different situations and have different informational needs.

By asking about the family situation and past experiences, the sonographer creates a space where the pregnant woman is invited to express her past experiences and expectations. We suggest that this is done to articulate the pregnant woman into a relationship through which knowledge and expectations can be managed and attuned. Accordingly, the sonographers attempt to reduce the gap between what is expected from undergoing an FTPRA and what might actually happen during the trajectory of the FTPRA. This is an important element for the realisation of an informed choice; it also serves the purpose of managing expectations.

One dimension in this mutual adjustment is the sonographer's attempt to manage the way in which a woman will react to a potential future message of being at high risk after the risk assessment has been done. A sonographer explains:

S4:   Before I start scanning I . . . emphasise that it is a risk assessment, which does not say anything about whether the fetus is diseased or not. I make sure I emphasise that the outcome is only a risk figure.

NS: Yes?

S4:   And then I say that the Danish Board of Health has made some guidelines, so if you receive a risk figure which is lower than 1 : 300, then you will continue pregnancy as usual. But if the risk figure is higher than 1 : 300, then we will talk about the possibility of undergoing extra examinations.

NS: Yes?

S4:   I emphasise that this does not mean that the fetus is necessarily diseased. If you make sure of emphasising this point, then only a few pregnant women will go into shock if they receive the message that they have received a risk which means that more examinations will be offered [high risk].

By making sure she tells the woman that the FTPRA is 'only' a risk assessment, the sonographer creatively attempts to manage the meaning of the message of being classified as 'high risk'. Below, a sonographer explains how she consciously tries to transform a risk figure which (according to the cut-off) is categorised as high risk into a positive result, which will give access to further testing possibilities. The sonographer reflects on how she has changed the language she used to frame risk results to the women:

S5:   When we started this programme, I described the two groups [below and above the cut-off point] as low risk and high risk, but today I make sure I do not say high risk any more.

NS: Why is that?

S5:   I think high risk sounds like an alarm bell and my experience is that they become unnecessarily nervous and upset if I use this category, so now I only describe the categories as two groups where one of the groups will lead to the positive offer of undergoing further examinations.

To protect the pregnant woman from unnecessary anxiety, the sonographer transforms the category of high risk into a positive message. Accordingly, the sonographer actively tries to manage the way in which the message will be understood in a potential future space of action and decision-making. If we look at these strategies of attunement in the light of the ideal of non-directiveness, understood as providing completely unbiased information, such strategies would be condemned as wrong or bad. The sonographer tries actively to engage in how risk will be understood and reacted upon in the future. However, this is not done with the aim of wanting the woman to act in specific ways but rather with the aim of protecting her from future emotional suffering in the case of being categorised as high risk.

Attuning life during ultrasound

Attuning knowledge and expectations is mentioned as a mode of doing good that has to be continuously attended to by the sonographer throughout the trajectory of the FTPRA. Another important dimension of this mode of doing good is the attunement of the meaning of the fetus through the practice of ultrasonography. At the point of pregnancy where an FTPRA is undertaken (weeks 11–13) the woman has rarely felt the fetus move. Many pregnant women say that that at this stage the pregnancy seems unreal (Schwennesen and Koch 2009). Seeing the image on the ultrasound screen, however, has the potential of escalating the social birth of the baby, thereby speeding up the creation of new identities of fetal subjecthood and maternal responsibility (Drapley 2002, Mitchell 2001, Taylor 2000, Sandelowski 1994, Schwennesen and Koch 2009). In interviews the sonographers reflect on how to be actively involved in the performance of the image on the screen in order to relate to the transformative effects it may have on the pregnant woman and her relationship to the fetus. A sonographer explained:

S3:   I have thought a lot about the fact that if a fetus ends up being categorised as high risk and if you, during ultrasound, have said that 'oh, this is sweet, there is a little arm there and you can hear the heart beat', then the woman will develop another relationship to the fetus, which is different if you have only seen pregnancy through a mark on a strip, right? During ultrasound you will both see it and hear it, right? Having seen it on a screen is different from knowing it intellectually. I think that we should not be too enthusiastic about how fantastic it is to see the fetus on the screen.

To be accountable for the possible future emerging in the case of high risk, the sonographers emphasise the importance of paying particular attention to their body language and which interpretation of the image they promote. Petchesky argues that ultrasound 'images by themselves lack "objective" meanings' (Petchesky 1987: 78) and therefore the different shades of grey emerging on the ultrasound screen need to be interpreted for the image to become meaningful in practice. This fundamental lack of meaning of ultrasound images provides a space in which different meanings of the image may be crafted during ultrasonography (Drapley 2002, Haraway 1997, Mitchell 2001, Schwennesen and Koch 2009). The sonographers explain how they try to accommodate their body language and the interpretation of the image on the screen to the emerging results in order to protect the pregnant woman from any future negative surprise. If during the scan the sonographer sees signs that a (problematic) high risk will be calculated, such as a large nuchal translucency or a nasal bone that is difficult to define, she will distance herself from the woman and not engage in any dialogue about what is seen on the ultrasound image. By doing so, she attempts not to contribute to the enactment of the image on the screen as a living child. Conversely, if the sonographer expects that a (non-problematic) low risk will be calculated, she will be more engaged in the enactment of the fetus as life by saying things like, 'this one is active' and 'this one is waving to you'. Such caring practices may be seen as strategies through which sonographers actively try to manage hope before, during and after ultrasound in order to shape the potential future space of decision-making in the case of a high-risk classification.

Second point of passage: communicating risk with care

What is articulated in the analysis above is a realisation that life and risk are not entities transmitted from the sonographer to the pregnant woman in a non-directive manner.

Instead, the meaning of life and risk evolves through a relationship of attunement, where the sonographer is actively and consciously involved. This process of meaning-making continues throughout the trajectory of the FTPRA where the next passage point is the situation where a risk figure is communicated and a decision has to be made on how to act on this basis. In the following we articulate a second mode of doing good as 'allowing resistance' in the clinical encounter of risk communication and decision-making.

The cut-off point and the regulatory framework of prevention

After the scan the pregnant woman must wait for the final risk result in the clinic's waiting area while the sonographer goes into another room where she types the result of the scan into a computer. Together with the data from the serum test, she calculates the overall risk result. The result of the test is presented to the pregnant woman as a risk figure on an infinite scale and it could be 1 : 50, 1 : 350 or 1 : 20,000. In cases where the risk figure is assessed as high according to a cut-off point (1 : 300), it will automatically open up a space of possible preventive action as it gives access to undergo an invasive test.

The cut-off point expresses a norm of effective prevention; it is settled on the basis of complex cost-benefit calculations made with the aim of defining a limit of access to invasive testing that most effectively distributes pregnancies into the categories of high risk (requiring an invasive test) and low risk (not requiring a test). This calculation is based on a large sample of epidemiological data (Nicolaides 2004) and expresses a relationship between the detection and false-positive rates and economic cost. There is a trade-off between these factors and where the exact limit is set is not objectively evident, but it is based on normative and political decisions balancing the different interests. The sonographers explain that they realise that the cut-off point might influence their own professional interpretation of a risk figure as either good or bad. One sonographer said:

> S6:   A figure is not just a figure. Working with prenatal testing within this framework makes me think that when a risk figure is around 1 : 300 then it is not a good situation. It is not nice for me to go out and deliver such a result.

This illustrates the way in which the cut-off point may regulate sonographers' interpretation of risk in certain ways. Latour (1987) developed the concept *immutable mobile* to capture the ways in which standards (cut-off points) are capable of translating interests across time and space. We may understand the cut-off point as such a standard, which may possibly transport the rationality of effective prevention into processes of decision-making.

Allowing resistance in processes of knowledge production

In interviews, sonographers acknowledge that they are placed in a powerful position, which involves an inevitable influence on how risk is understood. The challenge for the caring sonographer is, according to the sonographers (for instance, S4): 'not to force one's own view – or the institutional frameworks' opinion upon them, when you present them with the answer'. The sonographers describe practices of care as an art that requires empathy, obligingness, openness and a continuous judgement of the situation. A sonographer sums up the challenges she faces thus:

> S1:   You have to be careful not to make the process of the FTPRA too standardised, that you make sure to spend time on each person you are confronted with and come to understand their background and their expectations and their views and

then take a bearing on that, so that we do not misunderstand each other. This is an art, which sometimes succeeds and sometimes doesn't.

A number of social science scholars have studied the implications of an increasing use of risk in the context of pregnancy and prenatal testing (Ettorre 2002, Helén 2005, Lippman 1991, Lupton 1999, Weir 1996). While such scholars seem to emphasise the disciplining effects of risk knowledge and the control and constraints on action derived from such knowledge, professional practices of care open up possible ways in which the provision of risk knowledge might allow space for agency and the emergence of alternative notions of risk. Using the example of knowledge production in the context of animal experiments, Vinciane Despret makes a convincing argument about care and its relationship to the workings of power. She argues that power works, not as a deterministic force but through processes of mutual expectations and trust, which make entities available to emerging in particular ways (Despret 2004). In the context of animal experiments, the mutual relationship and expectations between the experimenter, the animal and the organiser of the experiment together determine what the animal is allowed to become (for example, dull or intelligent). In this regard, Despret describes the role of a caretaker as someone interested in the possible 'becoming' of identities in processes of knowledge production without steering into normative evaluations of how it should become. She contrasts the role of a caretaker with that of a judge or a master, who require docility from the entities through which knowledge is made (Despret 2004: 123). According to Despret, the possibility of 'resistance' in processes of knowledge production determines whether the setting produces passive or docile bodies or bodies that are cared for. If we apply this to the professional practice of the FTPRA, the task for the caring sonographer is to provide a space for the pregnant woman where she is allowed to act in unexpected ways and articulate alternative notions of risk. This requires attention to the specific pregnant woman and her particular situation, and a continuous openness to unexpected articulations and transformations of risk. This form of attunement and continuous situated awareness in the process of the FTPRA is particularly important if we take the transformative capabilities of an FTPRA into account. Several sonographers emphasise that a pregnant woman's notion of risk and wishes and values might change during the course of an FTPRA. The consultant says:

C1:   It might be that a pregnant woman and her partner attend an FTPRA with an idea that they will accept the offer of undergoing an invasive test if the fetus is classified as high risk. But in that situation they do not expect that they will receive a high risk, it is not what they expect or hope for when they come to us in the first place, right?

NS: Yes?

C1:   But that situation changes and their wishes might change too in the case of being classified as high risk and then we have to allow them to make another choice [of saying no to the offer], right?

NS: So you feel that the pregnant woman's wishes and values might change by undergoing an FTPRA?

C1:   Yes, that's for sure, yes!

The sonographer emphasises the importance of allowing a woman to change her mind during the course of undergoing an FTPRA. In such situations the challenge for the caring sonographer is to allow the pregnant woman to resist by understanding risk and acting in ways different from what is implicitly intended by the cut-off point or what the sonographer immediately would expect from her.

'What would you do, Doctor?' Situating influence in the context of uncertain knowledge
A particularly difficult situation for sonographers arises when a woman asks for their professional opinion. The sonographers' articulations of how to respond to such a question, reveal a third mode of doing good, which we express as 'situating influence'. According to the definition of non-directiveness by Rehmann-Sutter (2009), non-directiveness involves restraining oneself from giving practical advice. Thus, giving direct advice is considered off limits. A common expression from our interviews with pregnant women was their feeling of being left in limbo in the face of complex risk knowledge and their continuing search for tools that could be used to make the risk figure meaningful and thus actionable (Schwennesen *et al.* 2010). Below is an excerpt from an interview with a woman who received a risk of 1:164. During the interview she expressed the frustrations she felt when being told to make her own decision on the basis of what she considered a meaningless risk figure. In an attempt to make sense of how to act, the woman reacted, almost by reflex, by asking the health professional what she would do if she was in her situation. She said:

> I tried to talk to the sonographer who informed me about the risk. 'What would you do?' was my first question, right, 'What would you recommend me to do?' and she said that she could not tell me anything at all. But I felt immediately that I needed something to compare with. A number is just a number, right. I work with numbers all day and I know that you can perceive a number from 1000 different views, right, and it will mean something different every time.

This woman expressed a common frustration among women and partners having to make a decision on the basis of partial risk knowledge. While the official guidelines emphasise the ideals of non-directiveness and autonomy in decision-making and in so doing configure the relationship between professional and patients in the direction of patient authority, the pregnant woman seeks to reinstall authority in the sonographer by asking for advice. In doing so, the sonographer is re-authorised to act as a paternalistic expert and is asked to articulate her experienced advice. Authorisation refers here to a relationship where one party authorises another by communicating faith and trust in the ability of the other to act competently and in accordance with the expectations expressed by the first party (Despret 2004: 120). We might understand a pregnant woman's question such as 'What would you do in my situation?' as an attempt to avail herself of the sonographer's expert evaluation of the situation and as expressing a resistance to the delegated role of authority in processes of decision-making.

In describing to NS how she would tackle a situation where a pregnant woman asks for her advice, a sonographer (S2) explains: 'Usually I reply that I have never experienced such a situation myself and for that reason I do not know how I would react. You are the only one who can make such a decision'. With this reply, the sonographer acts 'correctly' according to the regulatory framework of non-directiveness, by resisting the authorisation of her as a paternalistic expert and in response installs the pregnant woman as an expert who has to make her decision herself according to her own values and needs. However, several sonographers express concern about not leaving a pregnant woman 'behind' and emphasise their obligation to provide her with meaning-making tools to navigate in the complex sea of information she is presented with. In this situation, caring for the pregnant woman by providing meaning-making tools and the ideal of non-directiveness seem to clash.

One sonographer (S1) explains how she tries to accommodate those two ideals by providing statistical data on how other women have reacted in the same situation. She says: 'I may tell them that most Danish citizens would do x, if they were in your situation: this is often helpful'. By making this selected statistical data available to the pregnant woman the sonographer attempts to support her in the process of creating existential footing and reaching a meaningful decision. In her view this strategy does not conflict with the ideal of non-directiveness. She says:

> S1:   This is only statistics . . . we know what people do and what they don't do. This is completely neutral knowledge and they can use it as they want: most people are happy with that.

For this sonographer, making statistical data available becomes a means through which she can both live up to the ideal of non-directiveness and accommodate the pregnant woman's request for professional influence and advice. This process occurs through a transformation of the understanding of what neutrality means. With this transformation she becomes able to guide the pregnant women in a fashion that does not violate the non-directiveness principle but, nevertheless, helps the pregnant woman to gain existential footing in the decision-making process.

The sonographer enacts knowledge as something that can and should be articulated responsibly to the particular pregnant woman to support her in her own decision-making, taking her particular situation into account. Another sonographer said:

> S4:   So you are placed in a very powerful position, but if you are aware of that, then you become able to differentiate the knowledge and use it to guide them through the decision-making process and help them to arrive at a place that you sense they will feel the happiest about, right?

This sonographer emphasises how she tries to use knowledge to support and guide the individual woman in her decision-making process. Whereas one could argue that such a form of conscious knowledge differentiation would work against the principle of non-directiveness and thus the possibility of the pregnant woman's ability to make an autonomous decision, such practices may be understood as exactly what makes decision-making possible in a situation where complex risk knowledge is experienced as basically meaningless. It illustrates a point from STS that individual reflexive action, such as choice, is possible only in a heterogeneous collective network (Callon and Law 1997).

If we acknowledge that meaningful decisions are made through interdependent relations, we suggest that a careful professional response to the question 'what would you do in my situation?' might be for sonographers to accept the authority which is trustingly delegated to them and provide pregnant women with situated influence or advice. This would represent a shared responsibility for the process of decision-making and the decision which is to be made. According to Despret, what makes the difference between requiring docility and giving care in such situations is the extent to which the pregnant woman is allowed to resist her allotted role and what is expected from her in the process and to act in unexpected ways, for instance, by challenging the advice given. We might conclude with Despret that 'to fulfil expectations, to be available to others' beliefs or concern is not *necessarily* [our italics] to obey these expectations or beliefs' (Despret 2004: 123). From this perspective, influence or advice may be seen as an act of care if the pregnant woman is simultaneously allowed to act in unexpected ways.

Conclusion

In the last three decades or so, ideals of autonomous choice and non-directiveness have increasingly been framed as obvious solutions to what is considered as the problem of paternalism and authoritarian power in past programmes of prenatal testing and counselling. The new Danish guidelines on prenatal testing constitute an exemplary way in which such ideals are increasingly dominant in current regimes of prenatal testing in European and American countries. Framing the problems and solutions about current regimes of prenatal testing through the lens of choice, however, tends to collapse the debate about how to do good in prenatal testing and counselling into questions evolving around issues such as how to make non-directive counselling possible and how to make sure that autonomous choices can really be made. Such questions rely on an image of knowledge as stable facts that can be transmitted in a value-neutral manner from professional to pregnant woman. It implies a model of communication where the relationship between professional and pregnant woman and her partner is (ideally) stripped of any socio-material interaction and presents the professional job as purely technical: the sonographer has only to reveal already existing facts and communicate them to the pregnant woman and her partner in a non-directive manner.

Whereas such a representationalist view on fact production operates with a static and essentialist view on facts, this study illustrates that notions of life and risk are made and managed through the sonographer's continuous and active engagement in the production of facts throughout FTPRA trajectories. Knowledge of life and risk is not transmitted from the sonographer to the pregnant woman in a non-directive manner but evolves through relationships of attunement, where the sonographer is actively and consciously involved. We have thus shown how the clinic is a site where medical knowledge is creatively produced in the clinical encounter rather than simply consumed (Latimer et al. 2006). This process is not predetermined, but needs to be approached as a relationship between the institutional framing of risk, the clinical organisation, the sonographer and the pregnant women's particular situation.

A gap between official ideals and practice is documented in the present study, in alignment with other studies (Anderson 1999, Hunt et al. 2005, Petersen 1999, Williams et al. 2002). Whereas such a gap has been described as a serious problem of oppressive power perhaps resulting in coercive moments of decision-making, this study opens up for 'modes of doing good care' as other, more practice-based, solutions to the 'problem of power' in prenatal counselling. We would like to emphasise three modes of doing good care which come to the fore in our study: (i) a continuous attunement of knowledge and expectations, (ii) providing space for allowing resistance in the process of prenatal knowledge production and decision-making, and (iii) providing situated influence in the context of uncertain and ambiguous knowledge and acceptance of a shared responsibility for the decision which is to be made, in situations where authority is trustingly delegated to the sonographers. Such modes are not compatible with the non-directive ethos but express ways of reducing emotional suffering and supporting a pregnant woman's ability to make meaningful choices on the basis of uncertain knowledge. In opposition to an ethics aiming at non-directiveness and autonomous decision-making, such modes of doing good care express an ethics of being locally accountable for the ways in which programmes of prenatal testing inevitably intervene in pregnant women's lives and of taking responsibility for the entities and phenomena that emerge through such knowledge production.

If we wish to relate to the question of how to do good in prenatal testing and decision-making, we must start from the premises that prenatal knowledge production is an intervention in the categories through which pregnant women come to experience themselves and their relationship to others and that decisions are made through interdependent practices (Struhkamp 2005). Accordingly, we have to draw our attention away from questions of correspondence (how to represent facts in an objective manner) towards questions of intervention, such as how to intervene in temporal knowledge production and decision-making with care. To be care-fully involved in processes of knowledge production, within an organisational and health political framework with multiple objectives such as prevention and choice, requires difficult and creative work. Such inventive creative work is rarely recognised as being valuable in current regimes of choice. This article is an attempt to articulate caring practices to make them available for recognition, appreciation and assessment as well as for critical reflection and discussion.

Acknowledgements

This article was written in partial fulfilment of a PhD project exploring the social implications of first trimester prenatal risk assessment in Denmark, which was funded by Bio-campus, research priority area, Copenhagen University. We thank Mette Nordahl Svendsen, Henriette Langstrup Nielsen and two anonymous reviewers for constructive comments on earlier drafts.

Notes

1 Non-directiveness has been increasingly criticised in professional literature on prenatal counseling (Weil *et al*. 2006) and has been complemented by the model of shared decision-making (Elwyn *et al*. 2000: 138). Despite the critique, non-directiveness continues to be the ethical gold standard against which professional practice is assessed.
2 See, for instance, the UK Human Genetics Commission (2006) report entitled 'Making babies: reproductive decisions and genetic technologies'.
3 The Fetal Medicine Foundation is a charity foundation headed by Professor Kypros Nicolaides that has developed an international training programme for conducting the FTPRA. See Fetal Medicine Foundation (2010).
4 In most cases the woman will attend the FTPRA together with her partner. In the following I focus on the woman and do not make visible the ways in which pregnant woman and their partners may experience the process of undergoing an FTPRA in different ways. See Drapley (2002) for an illustrative example of how gender plays a significant role for the experience of undergoing ultrasound.
5 The sonographers had the following years of experience. In order to maintain their anonymity their experience is listed in intervals: S1: 16–20 years, S2: 1–5 years, S3: 11–15 years, S4: 11–15 years, S5:6–10 years, S6: 6–10 years, C1: 10–15 years.

References

Anderson, G. (1999) Nondirectiveness in prenatal genetics: patients read between the lines, *Nursing Ethics*, 6, 2, 126–36.
Boltanski, L. and Thévenot, L. (1991) *De la Justifications. Les Économies de la Grandeur (On justification. The economies of grandeur)*. Paris: Editions Gallimard.

Brunger, F. and Lippman, A. (1995) Resistance and adherence to the norms of genetic counseling, *Journal of Genetic Counseling*, 4, 3, 151–67.

Callon, M. and Law, J. (1997) After the individual in society: lessons on collectivity from science, technology and society, *Canadian Journal of Sociology*, 22, 12, 165–82.

Clarke, A. (1997) The process of genetic counselling. In Harper, P. and Clarke, A. (eds) *Genetics, Society and Clinical Practice*. Oxford: BIOS Scientific Publishers.

Danish Board of Health (2004) *Nye retningslinjer for fosterdiagnostik (New guidelines for prenatal testing)*. Copenhagen: Danish Board of Health.

Despret, V. (2004) The body we care for: figures of anthropo-zoo-genesis, *Body and Society*, 10, 2–2, 111–34.

Drapley, J. (2002) 'It was a real good show': the ultrasound scan, fathers and the power of visual knowledge, *Sociology of Health & Illness*, 24, 2, 771–95.

Elwyn, G., Gray, J. and Clarke, A. (2000) Shared decision making and non-directiveness in genetic counselling, *Journal Medical Genetics*, 37, 2, 135–8.

Ettorre, E. (2002) *Reproductive Genetics, Gender and the Body*. London: Routledge.

Fetal Medicine Foundation (2010) Certificates of competence: the 11–13 week scan. Available at http://www.fetalmedicine.com/fmf/training-certification/certificates-of-competence/the-11-136-week-scan/ (last accessed 15 September 2010).

Foucault, M. (1978) *The History of Sexuality: an Introduction. Vol. 1*. New York: Pantheon.

Franklin, S. and Roberts, C. (2006) *Born and Made: An Ethnography of Preimplantation Genetic Diagnosis*. New Jersey: Princeton University Press.

Hacking, I. (1986) 'Making up people'. In Heller, T., Morton, S. and Wellbery, D. (eds) *Reconstructing Individualism. Autonomy, Individuality and the Self in Western Thought*. Stanford: Stanford University Press.

Haraway, D. (1997) *modest_witness@second_millennium.femaleman©Meets_OncoMouse™: Feminism and Technoscience*. New York: Routledge.

Harper, P.S. (2004) *Practical Genetic Counselling*. London: Arnold.

Harris, R., Lane, B., Harris, H., Williamson, P., *et al.* (1999) National confidential enquiry into counselling for genetic disorders by non geneticists: general recommendations and specific standards for improving care, *British Journal of Obstetrics and Gynaecology*, 106, 7, 658–63.

Helén, I. (2005) Risk management and ethics in antenatal care. In Bunton, R. and Petersen, A. (eds) *Genetic Governance. Health, Risk and Ethics in the Biotech Area*. London: Routledge.

Human Genetics Commission (2006) *Making Babies: Reproductive Decisions and Genetic Technologies*. London: HOC.

Hunt, L., Voogd, K.B. de and Castaneda, H. (2005) The routine and the traumatic in prenatal genetic diagnosis: does clinical information inform patient decision-making? *Patient Education and Counseling*, 56, 3, 302–12.

Latimer, J., Featherstone, K., Atkinson, P., Clarke, A., *et al.* (2006) Rebirthing the clinic. The interaction of clinical judgment and genetic technology in the production of medical science, *Science, Technology & Human Values*, 31, 5, 599–630.

Latour, B. (1987) *Science in Action*. Milton Keynes: Open University Press.

Law, J. (1994) *Organizing Modernity*. Oxford: Blackwell.

Lippman, A. (1991) Prenatal genetic testing and screening: constructing needs and reinforcing inequities, *American Journal of Law and Medicine*, 17, 1–2, 15–50.

Lupton, D. (1999) Risk and the ontology of pregnant embodiment. In Lupton, D. (ed.) *Risk and Sociocultural Theory: New Directions and Perspectives*. New York: Cambridge University Press.

Marteau, T.M., Dormandy, E. and Michie, S. (2001) A measure of informed choice, *Health Expectations*, 4, 2, 99–108.

Mitchell, L.M. (2001) *Baby's First Picture. Ultrasound and the Politics of Fetal Subjects*. Toronto: University of Toronto Press.

Mol, A. (2002) *The Body Multiple. Ontology in Medical Practice*. Durham: Duke University Press.

Mol, A. (2006) Proving or improving: on health care research as a form of self-reflection, *Qualitative Health Research*, 16 3, 405–14.

Mol, A. (2008) *The Logic of Care. Health and the Problem of Patient Choice*. London: Routledge.

Mol, A., Moser, I. and Pols, J. (2010) *Care in practice. On tinkering in clinics, homes and farms.* Bielefeld: Transcript.

Nicolaides, K.H. (2004) *The 11–13 Week Scan.* London: Fetal Medicine Foundation.

Petchesky, R. (1987) Foetal images. The power of visual culture in the politics of reproduction. In Stanworth, M. (ed.) *Reproductive Technologies: Gender, Motherhood and Medicine.* Minneapolis: University of Minnesota Press.

Petersen, A. (1999) Counseling the genetically 'at risk': the poetics and politics of 'non-directiveness', *Health, Risk & Society,* 1, 3, 253–65.

Pilnick, A. (2008) 'It's something for you both to think about': choice and decision making in nuchal translucency screening for Down's syndrome, *Sociology of Health & Illness,* 30, 4, 511–30.

Pols, J. (2003) Enforcing patient rights or improving care? The interference of two modes of doing good in mental health care, *Sociology of Health & Illness,* 25, 4, 320–47.

Rapp, R. (2000) *Testing Women, Testing the Fetus: the Social Impacts of Amniocentesis in America.* New York: Routledge.

Rehmann-Sutter, C. (2009) Allowing agency. An ethical model of communicating personal genetic information. In Rehmann-Sutter, C. and Muller, H. (eds) *Disclosure Dilemmas in Ethics of Genetic Prognosis After the 'Right to Know/Not to Know' Debate.* Farnham: Ashgate.

Rothman, B.K. (1986) *The Tentative Pregnancy. Prenatal Diagnosis and the Future of Motherhood.* New York: Viking Penguin.

Sandelowski, M. (1994) Separate, but less unequal: fetal ultrasonography and the transformation of expectant mother/fatherhood, *Gender & Society,* 8, 2, 230–45.

Schwennesen, N. (2011) *Practicing Informed Choice. Inquiries into the Redistribution of Life, Risk and Relations of Responsibility in Prenatal Decision Making and Knowledge Production.* Centre for medical science and technology studies, Institute of public health, University of Copenhagen.

Schwennesen, N. and Koch, L. (2009) Calculating and visualizing life: matters of fact in the context of prenatal risk assessment. In Bauer, S. and Wahlberg, A. (eds) *Contested Categories. Life Science in Society.* Farnham: Ashgate.

Schwennesen, N., Koch, L. and Svendsen, M.N. (2009) Practising informed choice: decision making and prenatal risk assessment – the Danish experience. In Rehmann-Sutter, C. and Müller, H. (eds) *Disclosure Dilemmas. Ethics of Genetic Prognosis after the 'Right to Know/Not to Know' Debate.* Farnham: Ashgate.

Schwennesen, N., Svendsen, M.N. and Koch, L. (2010) Beyond informed choice: prenatal risk assessment, decision making and trust, *Clinical Ethics,* 5, 4, 207–16.

Struhkamp, R., Mol, A. and Swierstra, T. (2009) Dealing with In/dependence: doctoring in physical rehabilitation practice, *Science, Technology & Human Values,* 34, 1, 55–76.

Struhkamp, R.M. (2005) Patient autonomy: a view from the kitchen, *Medicine, Health Care and Philosophy,* 8, 1, 105–14.

Tabor, A., Philip, J., Madsen, M., Bang, J., *et al.* (1986) Randomised controlled trial of genetic amniocentesis in 4,606 low-risk women, *Lancet,* 327, 8493, 1287–96.

Taylor, J.S. (2000) Of sonograms and baby prams: prenatal diagnosis, pregnancy and consumption, *Feminist Studies,* 26, 2, 391–418.

Tørring, N., Jølving, L.R., Petersen, O.B.B., Holmskov, A., *et al.* (2008) Prænatal diagnostik i Århus og Viborg Amter efter implementering af første trimester-risikovurdering, *Ugeskrift for læger,* 170, 1, 50–4.

Webster, A. (2007) Crossing boundaries. Social science in the policy room, *Science, Technology & Human Values,* 32, 4, 458–78.

Weil, J., Ormond, K., Peters, J., Peters, K., *et al.* (2006) The relationship of nondirectiveness to genetic counseling: report of a workshop at the 2003 NSGC annual education conference, *Journal of Genetic Counseling,* 15, 2, 85–93.

Weir, L. (1996) Recent developments in the government of pregnancy, *Economy and Society,* 25, 3, 373–92.

Williams, C., Alderson, P. and Farsides, B. (2002) Is nondirectiveness possible within the context of antenatal screening and testing? *Social Science & Medicine,* 54, 3, 17–25.

'Wakey wakey baby': narrating four-dimensional (4D) bonding scans

Julie Roberts

Introduction

The aim of this essay is to explore the construction of meaning during four-dimensional (4D) ultrasound scans in the specific context of commercial 'bonding scans'. Although ultrasound in pregnancy has been an important research field for feminists, to date the limited scholarly literature around non-diagnostic ultrasound services has not engaged with the practice of ultrasound and social exchanges within the scan room, nor have we yet adequately explored the specificity of 4D technology. This new social practice of non-diagnostic or bonding scans prompts a reconsideration of ultrasound in practice. It has been widely claimed that 3- and 4D ultrasound imagery requires little or no expert interpretation. For example, I have argued elsewhere that, within the latest UK debates about the gestational time limit for abortion, lay people have been encouraged, even morally obligated, to view the latest fetal images in order to make informed contributions to the debate (Palmer 2009a). Here I describe a process of 'collaborative coding' in which sonographers and expectant parents work together to narrate the 3/4D scan imagery produced during a 'bonding scan'. I argue that this indicates that far from being self-evident, 3/4D imagery relies just as heavily on social interaction and discourse to be meaningful. However, there is some evidence that expectant parents are 'learning to see' for themselves and mobilising family knowledge and embodied experience in order to narrate the imagery on the screen in a way that is both socially and personally meaningful. In this sense, within the new social practice of 4D 'bonding scans', we see continuities with the performance of 2D ultrasound scans in antenatal care, but also new visual materials with which to construct social and family narratives. First, I provide an overview of the feminist literature to date around routine obstetric ultrasound in the clinical context and the role of sonographers and parents in making the imagery and the experience meaningful. I introduce the practice of 'bonding scans' in more detail and the small body of scholarly literature pertaining to non-diagnostic scans. I then describe the methods employed in the study reported here before moving on to the analysis.

The Sociology of Medical Screening, First Edition. Edited by Natalie Armstrong and Helen Eborall.
Chapters © 2012 The Authors. Book Compilation © 2012 Foundation for the Sociology of Health & Illness / Blackwell Publishing Ltd. Published 2012 by Blackwell Publishing Ltd.

Background

The routine use of obstetric ultrasound in antenatal care has transformed the experience of pregnancy for women in many parts of the world (Duden 1993, Sandelowski 1994b). Feminists have critiqued the use of ultrasound technology for medicalising pregnancy (Oakley 1984), for erasing pregnant women from view (Petchesky 1987, Stabile 1994, Mehaffy 2000), while constructing the fetus as patient and citizen (Franklin 1991, Berlant 1994, Casper 1998), and for devaluing women's embodied knowledge in favour of the technological and the visual (Sandelowski 1994b, Henwood 2001). Yet, women and their families report finding ultrasound examinations pleasurable (Petchesky 1987, Garcia *et al.* 2002). So long as the pregnancy is confirmed as healthy, women report that the scan is reassuring, that it confirms the reality of the pregnancy and provides an opportunity to 'meet' the baby (Clement *et al.* 1998, Bricker *et al.* 2000, Garcia *et al.* 2002).

Among sociological, feminist and anthropological studies, routine obstetric ultrasound scanning has long been recognised as a 'hybrid practice' (Taylor 1998): both medical and social meanings are incorporated into routine clinical practice as evidenced by, for example, the few minutes taken by sonographers at the end of a scan to obtain a take-home picture for the expectant parents, or the provision of an extra monitor so that women can watch the scan. Ultrasound is central to prenatal testing but is also used to produce 'baby's first picture' (Mitchell 2001). The boundaries between the medical and the social components of any scan are shifting, indistinct and permeable (Mitchell 2001), and perhaps ultimately impossible to disentangle (van Dijck 2005). Clinicians and patients have different attitudes and expectations of ultrasound examinations (Sandelowski 1994a) and the social and clinical elements are often in tension (Mitchell 2001, Taylor 2008): the clinical elements intrude on the social pleasures of scanning and the social expectations of scanning disrupt its clinical aims.

Sonograms are semiotic objects, with multiple and shifting meanings that vary by context but are also culturally and historically specific (Mitchell and Georges 1997). Sonographers are central to both clinical and social interpretation of ultrasound images. Mitchell argues that the sonographer's role is to translate ultrasound echoes into meaningful clinical data (percentages, numbers, statements of normality and abnormality), but also into socially meaningful data about maternal and fetal selfhood: all scans are 'acts of "translation" or "coding" in which technologically produced signs (reflected echoes) are translated into meaningful statements about the world' (Mitchell 2001: 108). While some of this translation work, according to Mitchell, is achieved through ongoing historical and social processes (such as routine use of ultrasound, wide dissemination of sonograms), it also takes place within the scan room. In the British National Health Service (NHS), this usually happens at the end of a routine appointment. After the measurements are recorded, the sonographer will take a few minutes to show the fetus to patients, helping them to see the 'baby' on the screen and trying to obtain a take-home picture. These take-home pictures are different from the clinically-necessary views, showing, for example, the profile of the fetus rather than femur length. Sonographers commonly guide their patients to make sense of the image on the screen, offer reassurances, and begin to construct fetal personhood, even as they complete the measurements necessary to prenatal testing and search for anomalies that may undermine claims to fetal personhood. Mitchell argues that women are heavily dependent on sonographers' accounts of the images on the screen 'in order to see their baby amidst the swirling grey mass of echoes' (Mitchell 2001: 120; see also Sandelowski 1994b), but, nonetheless, she acknowledges 'translation' is not a one-way process, with patients as passive recipients of expert knowledge, rather meaning emerges from the social interactions in the scan room. Women and their partners often interact with the screen as they would with a new born baby, admiring it, talking about it as a baby, and even talking to the image (Sandelowski 1994b, Mitchell 2001, Draper 2002). To a great extent, this interaction is dictated by norms and conventions and policed by sonographers who look for signs of 'good' parenting in these displays (Mitchell 2001).

Fetal imaging and images are the sites of complex struggles over meaning and over who has the authority to define the meaning of the technology and the images produced. This is evident in the public domain, where fetal images have been central to debates around abortion (Franklin 1991, Palmer 2009a). In the context of antenatal care, there is concern among the medical professions about women imposing their own interpretations on the function and significance of ultrasound. Clinicians fear that women may not be giving informed consent to prenatal screening but attending appointments because they want to 'see the baby' and they may not have necessarily thought about the information they might receive from the tests (Ockleford et al. 2003, Smith et al. 2004). Parents may instead use the scan as an opportunity to admire and get acquainted with the baby, to get baby's first picture, to involve their male partners in the pregnancy, to see the baby and for reassurance (Sandelowski 1994a, Mitchell 2001, Draper 2002, Gudex et al. 2006).

Bonding scans
Commercial 'keepsake' ultrasound services were first identified by the Food and Drug Agency in Texas in 1994 (Tanne 2004), and services are now also widely available in Europe, including the UK, the Netherlands, and Denmark. Companies offer a 4D scan in real-time, observed on a large LCD screen, and recorded to DVD, usually with a soundtrack of the client's choice. A number of still images are saved and subsequently printed on glossy paper, perhaps framed or transferred to key rings and other keepsakes. Such scans usually take place between 20 and 32 weeks' gestation when the fetus has developed to look more 'baby-like' but is still small enough to be imaged clearly. My focus here is on commercial ultrasound scanning services where the primary purpose is not diagnostic: variously termed 'keepsake fetal ultrasound' (Voelker 2005), 'boutique fetal imaging' (Chervenak 2005) and 'bonding scan' (a term used by a number of UK companies: Babybond, Insight Ultrasound, Preview Ultrasound and others). Such scans do not repeat clinical measurements and tests which are part of routine antenatal care, but provide a longer and more relaxed period of time in which to view the fetus. The stated purpose varies from 'seeing' the baby and getting some pictures to improved bonding and reassurance.

In the UK, bonding scans exist alongside the routine ultrasound scans offered by the National Health Service (NHS) at no cost to women. Women are offered two 2D scans as part of their routine antenatal care: a first scan at 10 to 13 weeks for dating the pregnancy and a second scan at 20 weeks for the detection of anomalies (National Collaborating Centre for Women's and Children's Health 2003: 10). While routine use of ultrasound in antenatal care is debated in some quarters (because of doubts about clinical effectiveness and concerns about the potential harm caused by the heating effects of ultrasound (Bricker et al. 2000), as well as evidence that women often do not have a full understanding of ultrasound or give informed consent (Garcia et al. 2002, Thorpe et al. 1993)), the appropriateness of using ultrasound for non-diagnostic purposes is more controversial. Women self-refer for commercial scans and are under no obligation to report the scan to their healthcare provider. Three- and four-dimensional technology is not used in routine antenatal care, because of limited utility (Kurjak et al. 2007) and therefore expectant parents seeking 3/4D images must turn to the commercial sector. The UK is less familiar with direct-to-consumer advertising of medical products and services than the USA, for example, but a range of services have entered the marketplace, including cosmetic surgery and 'health check' CT scans for the 'worried well' (Chrysanthou 2002). The market for non-diagnostic scans has rapidly expanded in the UK since 3/4D ultrasound became widely available (around 2003/4). Commercial scan providers must maintain a delicate balance between medical skill and the non-diagnostic functions of scanning. They must convince clients of their competence and safe practice, but also offer a different kind of experience that is additional to NHS antenatal care and screening (and thus worth paying for). Companies stress that they do not replace the anomaly scan and tread a careful line in order to both emphasise their medical authority and distance themselves from NHS scanning (which their clients often describe as stressful and frustratingly brief).

The critical response to 'bonding scans' from obstetrics, midwifery and related professions focuses on several core issues: the safety of additional exposure to ultrasound waves; the expertise of sonographers in the private sector; and disputed claims that ultrasound benefits maternal-fetal bonding (see for examples, Tanne 2004, Beech 2005, Chervenak 2005, Voelker 2005, Watts 2007).There are no specific regulations in the UK for controlling exposure to ultrasound although medical products are required to comply with the Medical Devices Regulations 2002 and guidance is issued by a number of professional bodies including the British Medical Ultrasound Society (Health Protection Agency 2010). Many professional bodies advise against extended exposure for 'keepsake' pictures, although they often acknowledge that evidence of biological risk is limited (British Medical Ultrasound Society 2007, ISUOG Bioeffects and Safety Committee et al. 2002). Similarly, concerns about who is offering commercial scans are fuelled by the knowledge that 'sonographer' is not yet a protected title (although this is under review; Lee and Paterson 2004, The Society and College of Radiographers 2009). The claim that ultrasound can enhance maternal-fetal bonding has been widely accepted within and beyond medicine but, in relation to non-diagnostic scanning, this claim is more commonly contested. The 'theory of ultrasound bonding' (Taylor 2008) was first proposed in the early 1980s and there continues to be disagreement about whether 'bonding' can be defined as a medically sanctioned justification for scanning and particularly for extended exposure to ultrasound waves (Taylor 2008). These debates are often encapsulated in calls for ultrasound to be restricted to its 'proper' (medical) use. More research is needed to understand how criticisms of 'bonding scans' relate to women's wellbeing and whether some of the criticisms are emerging from 'territorial' concerns about the control of ultrasound technology (Brezinka 2010). Considering 'bonding scans' within a longer history of critical engagement with ultrasound, it seems clear that the technology cannot be 'purified', cannot be 'purged of its cumbersome nonmedical (emotional, cultural) connotations' (van Dijck 2005) but rather needs to be understood as a 'hybrid practice' (Taylor 1998) and the meaning of ultrasound images as socially constructed within local and global contexts.

A small number of feminist scholars have engaged with the availability of non-diagnostic ultrasound services. José van Dijck (2005) has noted the flourishing of 'ultrasound-for-fun clinics' in the Netherlands, where typically second trimester scans are only offered in medical emergencies and sonographers are unregulated by the State. Gammeltoft and Nguyên (2007) describe the 'avid' consumption of ultrasound, including 4D scans, in Hanoi, Vietnam. Taylor describes the wide availability of 'entertainment ultrasound' or 'keepsake ultrasound' in the US as exemplary of 'a problematic nexus of medicine and consumerism' (Taylor 2008: 146), which is, in turn, implicated in reproductive politics. She critically examines the condemnation of non-diagnostic scans from professional bodies, noting the contested boundaries between the medical and 'entertainment' uses of ultrasound, and presents interviews with two ultrasound entrepreneurs about how they see their business. Taylor describes the use of 3/4D ultrasound by 'pregnancy crisis centres' seeking to use the striking imagery, and the potential effects on bonding, to dissuade women from terminating pregnancies. Kroløkke (2010) presents an analysis of the marketing websites of companies offering non-diagnostic, 4D scans in the USA and Denmark. She finds the tone of the marketing celebrates the technology and presents 4D ultrasound as an opportunity for empowerment and pleasure for women. The quality of the image, according to Kroløkke, makes it possible for women to be positioned as 'coparticipants' in the scan, rather than relying on sonographers to interpret grainy images, and allows the possibility of 'collective spectatorship'. Women are positioned as both consumers and tourists of their pregnancy. Finally, in a previous article, I have described the imaging of the placenta and umbilical cord in the process of 4D scans. I have argued that these structures are discursively constructed as obstructions to getting a 'good' picture of the fetus, and where possible they are deleted or ignored, but they may also be representations of the expectant mother on the screen (Palmer 2009b).

The study

This article is drawn from a wider study about the social and cultural meanings of sonograms (Palmer 2007). The study reported here builds on previous ethnographic research into clinical ultrasound scanning but focuses on 3/4D ultrasound and non-diagnostic scanning. This approach makes it possible to explore the social elements of the practice of scanning in more detail and to attend to the specificities of 3/4D technology. There are two key considerations here. First, the shift to 3/4D may represent a shift in the power to interpret images from sonographer to client. However, as I will show, 4D images are not as easy to interpret as we might expect. Second, 3/4D ultrasound produces images with new clarity and detail and visualises for the first time fetal facial 'expressions'. Therefore, this study is able to add to the literature by showing how clients and sonographer narrate these elements of the image.

The data were collected during an observational study of 'bonding scans'. Observations were carried out at three locations belonging to two UK companies between April and June 2006. The two companies were selected because they were very different in size and length of establishment. Data were collected in three geographically dispersed locations within the UK: one in the North West, one in the East Midlands and one in the South East. At each site, I spent whole days at the studios, speaking informally with staff and observing scans. The company directors gave consent to participate in the study. Consent was also sought from individual sonographers working at the company on observation days. All women presenting for 4D scans were approached and asked to participate. Consent was specifically sought from women clients, partners and family members who attended the scan appointment. Women received an information sheet, including information about how to contact the researcher with any future concerns. Informed consent was obtained from women in the waiting area, before the scan began. I observed 25 4D scans in total, each lasting 20–45 minutes. I observed five sonographers work across the three studios. Extensive field notes were taken in the scan room, focusing on clients' and sonographers' discussions around the imagery on the screen but also describing the environment of the scan room. Field notes were transcribed and anonymised.

Field notes for each scan were reviewed and compared. Transcripts were coded with recurrent categories that emerged from the data. The themes are presented here as components of a process of 'collaborative coding': that is to say the ways in which sonographers, pregnant women, and their accompanying guests narrate the imagery that they see on the screen. Below, I start by describing the beginning of a typical scan, and the role of the sonographer as expert guide. Then I describe a more collaborative process of making sense of the ultrasound imagery that emerged as the clients became more involved. Within this process of collaborative coding, the major themes are presented separately, divided into family resemblance, fetal personality, voicing the fetus, and mapping seeing and feeling.

The sonographer's role as expert guide

The lights are dimmed and a big, expensive-looking screen glows on the wall. The sonographer settles the pregnant woman on the couch, with her abdomen exposed, and covers her clothes with a towel before applying the transducing gel. Her partner (if present, or sometimes her mother), is encouraged to sit in the chair next to her and other guests can be settled on the sofa. The sonographer sits in front of the machine, looking at her own smaller screen with her back to the screen on the wall. Working in black-and-white 2D at first the sonographer takes a sweeping look at the fetus and begins to point out key landmarks to the clients; the heartbeat, proof of fetal life, is almost always the first thing pointed out:

> Sonographer: There's a strong heartbeat there, look . . . the baby is lying on its tummy . . . Feet over this side . . . head here.

The sonographer might also point out other internal organs (bladder, stomach) or the spine. If the clients want to know the sex of the baby, or if they want to confirm it, then this will be done next, all in 2D:

> Sonographer: Looking right between the legs there . . . looks like a girl.
> Sonographer: Looking for the million dollar question . . . it's a boy.

Then the sonographer begins to work to find the best angle for the transducer and, when she has a clear view of the face, with plenty of fluid around, changes to 4D in what looks like a simple flick of a switch. The sonographer starts the recording and guides the clients around the screen:

> Sonographer: This is a shoulder, elbow, the arm is bent up here . . . the face is turned away from us into the placenta.

The identification of limbs and face helps expectant parents get their bearing in the screen space. Descriptions of the screen may range from matter of fact labelling to more imaginative annotations, with the latter being very common, and including acting out the 'pose' of the fetus: for example, as a fetus raised a finger in front of its mouth, one sonographer drew the clients' attention to this by acting out the pose and adding a sound, 'shhh'.

Sometimes, the visual presence of the umbilical cord or placenta might require explanation as it is visually unfamiliar to most. I have argued elsewhere that these features of maternal anatomy are commonly described as either an obstacle to imaging, getting in the way of the 'camera' or as a representation of the expectant-mother on the screen (Palmer

2009b). This is an important link with feminist scholarship that has extensively critiqued the erasure of the female body from public fetal images (Duden 1993, Stabile 1994, Taylor 1998, Mehaffy 2000), but I do not intend to explore this theme further here except to note that the appearance of the placenta or umbilical cord often requires sonographers to mobilise their clinical expertise, for example to offer reassurance that these structures are located appropriately. The ability to recognise these structures and to reassure clients in a professional and authoritative manner is a necessary part of the role: here is a moment when the boundaries between medical and 'bonding' scans are explicitly blurred.

Collaborative coding

Ultrasound clients soon begin to learn their way around the screen and to take a more active role in coding the imagery on the screen, hesitantly at first ('is that a foot?'), then becoming more confident ('look, you can see his little mouth moving'). Bonding scans are often attended by partners, children, other family members and friends and any number of observers might join in the construction of a narrative. While this can be enjoyable, even 4D scans can be surprisingly difficult to read. Some clients find it upsetting if they cannot make any sense of the image on the screen, especially pregnant women, and especially when other observers are describing what they see and they have to admit 'I can't see anything!' I saw this happen more than once, although in each case the sonographer was able to orientate the woman to the image and, in time, she began to make out the fetus on the screen.

However, this collaborative coding is not just a question of confidence or competency in making sense of the images on the screen. The participation of the pregnant women and family members is necessary to making the narration more personalised. The sonogram is annotated in such a way as to make it both socially and personally meaningful. That is to say that sonographers can actively construct the visualised fetus as 'baby', drawing on visible markers of personhood and generic ideals of 'cuteness', but family members can make specific connections with family identity and history, annotating familiar facial features and behaviours, and 'weaving the fetus into a network of kinship relations' (Mitchell 2001: 134). The following subsection describes the process of collaboratively coding the imagery in detail.

Remarking resemblance: making connections
A 4D scan gives expectant parents new information about the appearance and behaviour of the fetus in the womb, and this information can be used to start to make connections between the existing family and the new baby. Previous studies concerning 2D ultrasound have found that the sonographer draws attention to anatomical features to construct fetal personhood, these have notably been interior structures, such as the spine, bladder, heart and brain, although (skeletal) fingers and toes have also been important synecdoches for the 'baby' (Mitchell 2001). With 4D imaging, surface features are rendered visible and as such become more significant. Particular points of connection are found in physical appearance, pose and, deduced from these, personality. The observation of these family resemblances are often very touching and sentimental, but can also be irreverent. Expectant parents, seeing one another in the baby, may turn and say:

Pregnant woman: She's got your nose.
    Male partner: I think she's got your mouth.

These comments may be accompanied by a gentle touch. One woman stroked her partner's brow as she commented upon the baby's likeness to his father in this regard. However, these comments about appearance are not always so reverent. Many people taunted one another with good-humoured insults:

> Pregnant woman: He's better looking than you anyway! (to her male partner).
> Male partner: She's got my nose.
> Family member: As long as she hasn't got your ears!

Such comments might also be self-deprecating rather than directed to others, with expectant parents hoping not to burden their children with some aspect of their own appearance that they dislike, or taking responsibility for some 'undesirable' feature such as 'big feet'. In rare cases, ultrasound imagery may help make disconnections: for example, one pregnant woman was relieved to see that the fetus did not resemble its biological father. She was very concerned to comment on the facial features that were like her own and comforted to see that the biological father's most striking facial features could not be seen in the baby. However, family resemblance is not always about physical appearance, but can be found in position and pose. A fetus, imaged with arms raised and hands visible to the side of the face, perhaps 'snuggling' into the placenta, may draw the comment: 'I sleep like that' or 'Ellen sleeps like that' (referring to a sibling). In this way, resemblance is constructed from pose or behaviour rather than purely from appearance. While the annotation of family resemblance with ultrasound images has been observed with 2D scans (Mitchell 2001), the latest 4D technology arguably strengthens the possibility of this kind of narration, since surface facial features are shown in new detail. Websites advertising 4D scans often display 'before' and 'after' (birth) photographs to demonstrate the similarity in appearance (Kr"løkke 2010). The capacity to preview the baby's appearance is one selling point of 4D ultrasound.

Fetal personality
Resemblance is also described in terms of personality. The baby may be described as 'shy' (difficult to image), or 'not shy' (easy to image), with the connection to one or other parent: 's/he's like me'. The baby may be seen as sleepy and laid back, or active and 'on the go', and similar comparisons made. Similar arm movements may be described as 'waving', 'punching' or 'swimming'. A fetus with arms up to its face might be described as 'hiding', or a more aggressive interpretation might be made: 'he's going to be a martial artist'. Hands near the nose and mouth might be irreverently described as the baby picking its nose, or more sentimentally described as baby 'blowing a kiss'. The two comments may even comfortably co-exist in the same portion of conversation, suggesting the temporary and fluid nature of these kinds of interpretations. Mitchell (2001) has described a similar process of coding movement on the (2D) screen in terms of fetal subjectivity and personality.

As in Mitchell's (2001) description, all parties in the scan room cooperate to interpret the imagery on the screen:

> Pregnant woman: Sleepy girl . . . did she open her eyes then? . . . wow!
> Sonographer: She's settled down again now . . . see her mouth going? She's got her hands in front of her face . . . there's a little smile . . . it's all too much. She's put her thumb in her mouth.
> Male partner: She's sucking her thumb (laughing).

In this exchange, three adults cooperate in making the images on the screen meaningful. The imaginative interpretations consist of a collaborative coding of the imagery, whereby an interpretation made by one observer is picked up and repeated, moderated or expanded upon by another. In this example, hands near the face and a few movements of the mouth are narrated to create an impression of a sleepy, comfortable and contented baby. The sonographer begins the theme, but it is taken up by both expectant parents and becomes a mutually acceptable interpretation of the images on the screen

Fetal facial expressions, imaged for the first time with 3/4D technology, are used to help build a picture of fetal personality, as clients identify smiles, frowns, yawns, 'thoughtful' expressions and more:

> Pregnant woman: Aah he's having a smile.
>   Male partner: He's laughing.
>   Sonographer: They do laugh.
>   Observer: He's enjoying the music!

In this playful exchange, all four adults envision a happy and good-humoured baby. The background music that plays in the room as it is recorded to the scan DVD is incorporated into the narrative and the facial movements on the screen narrated as a positive reaction to this external stimulus. However, it is not only happy facial expressions that are commented upon. 'Grumpy' and 'serious' faces are also described.

A 'little frowny face' can be just as endearing as a smiley one, and the tone of the commentary can be gently mocking, as if talking about a small child who is not seriously unhappy, only play-acting an exaggerated sulk.

Speaking to and for the fetus
Also comparable with Mitchell's (2001) study, many people spoke to the screen, with varying degrees of self-consciousness and seriousness, commonly addressing the fetus with instructions and greetings:

> Pregnant woman: Wakey wakey baby.
>   Male partner: Hello.
>   Sonographer: Turn this way, little tinker.

This 'interaction' with the fetus on the screen as if it is the baby is arguably one way in which expectant parents begin to create an identity for the new baby. By addressing the fetus, they prefigure a new individual and family member. They playfully imagine that the fetus can conceptualise the outside world looking in, adding credence to the interpretation of fetal movements as intentional and socially meaningful.

It is common to give the fetus a voice, speaking on the baby's behalf, to narrate the process of the scan and the fetus' imagined experience of it:

> Pregnant woman: Who's doing that?
> Pregnant woman: They're looking at me.
> Pregnant woman: It's squished in here!

The interaction is imagined to be two-sided, as if the fetus is aware of the scan taking place and of observers looking on. It is difficult to explain the status of these kinds of remarks. Mitchell argues that neither expectant parents nor sonographers view these kinds of 'interactions' as a joke, but rather 'an enjoyable form of interaction or contact with the fetus that ultrasound makes possible' (2001: 134).

Perhaps we should not look for an unambiguous understanding of these remarks but remember that: 'The virtual fetus both is *and* isn't "real" and necessarily, therefore, constructs a conflicted spectator' (Mehaffy 2000: 190). However, imaginative narratives also serve a purpose within the commercial scanning experience. Sonographers are very aware of the limitations of the technology and the high expectations of clients. They often expressed a feeling of being 'dependent on', even 'at the mercy of', the fetus, needing an appropriate position, a relatively still fetus, and plenty of fluid around the face. The difficulties of getting a clear scan picture are often explained by reference to the 'personality' of the fetus, rather than in technical terms. Fetuses are very often described as awkward and uncooperative. Sonographers speak to the fetus as if to a young child who won't stay still for their photo to be taken: 'She's a little tinker'. A fetus that is glimpsed but proves difficult to image clearly is described as 'teasing me', or 'playing peek-a-boo'. This is frustrating but these difficulties can also be a source of amusement. In several scans that I observed where the fetus consistently returned its hands to a position in front of its face, it became a source of fun. Despite the frustrations and the various measures that it necessitated to try and get some clear images (going for a walk, eating sugary foods, changing position), the clients seemed amused and delighted, especially as the difficulties were coupled with a commentary that described the fetus' behaviour in terms of 'hiding', 'being shy' or 'playing peek-a-boo'. The frustrations of the process are mitigated by the cute and charming interpretations, which often successfully keep clients content and engaged even if 'baby isn't cooperating'. While similar descriptions of 'uncooperative babies' are found in clinically-driven scanning (Mitchell 2001), here the aim of the scan is different, and this along with the commercial element perhaps exaggerates the need to manage 'difficult' scans in a way that eases the social interaction.

Mapping seeing and feeling

Ultrasound gives pregnant woman information about the fetus that may complement or conflict with their embodied knowledge of the fetus. Feminist scholars have described the conflict that sometimes arises between technological and embodied knowledge of pregnancy in the clinical context, arguing that technological information, and particularly visual evidence, tends to be more highly valued by clinicians and sometimes male partners (Sandelowski 1994b, Henwood 2001, Draper 2002). My observations suggest that, rather than becoming disembodied spectators, women actively engage in a process of relating the images on the screen to their own bodies, and also involve their partners in recognising this relationship between image and body.

I was struck by how often I observed women looking back and forth between the screen and their own bodies as if trying to locate the image inside them. The size of the fetus was a common concern. Most companies use a large LCD screen on the wall, and at one clinic the images are projected onto a white wall, and women often asked 'So how big is the baby now?' or 'Does it look big to you?'. A momentary anxiety is caused by the size of the baby on the screen, and sonographers must dispel it quickly. Women also asked how the screen relates to their body:

Pregnant woman: So the baby's head is this side, yeah?
Pregnant woman: It's that far up, is it? (looking at where the transducer is
            positioned).
Pregnant woman: Is she lying across me at the moment?

Sometimes there is a sense of disorientation, perhaps when the sensations do not easily correspond with the visual information:

Pregnant woman: It's weird seeing it and feeling it.

One excited father-to-be on seeing movement on the screen asks:

Male partner: Can you feel that?

And his partner answers uncertainly:

Pregnant woman: No . . . oh . . . I probably can feel that.

For some women, the visual helped make sense of physical sensations. One woman described feeling a lot of pressure on one side of her body. She had imagined this to be hands or feet but found that it was probably the fetus' bottom, at least on this particular day. The scan was often an opportunity for the woman and her partner to share information and, in a sense, compare experiences. Some male partners were keen to observe movement on the screen and then check back with their pregnant partner about the corresponding sensation:

Male partner: He's stretching, can you feel that?

It was also a chance for women to convey their experiences to their partners in new ways. One woman, observing the amazement of her male partner at the 4D imagery says:

Pregnant woman: See! You have to believe me now when I say that she is kicking me!

These observations suggest that a 'bonding scan' is not a purely visual experience and that the imagery on the screen does not always remain 'out there', disembodied, obscuring pregnant women from view, but can provide a means to confirm or explain sensations felt by the pregnant woman and help communicate these to partners and family members. Nonetheless, some discursive work is required to map the distant, and massively enlarged, image onto the pregnant body.

Conclusions

This essay has described the practice of 4D 'bonding scans' and a process of 'collaborative coding' in which sonographers and expectant parents work together to narrate the imagery on the screen. Previous studies have identified obstetric ultrasound as a 'hybrid practice' (Taylor 1998), in which sonographers and patients construct social meaning from the imagery on the screen. Researchers have found that women rely heavily on sonographers to interpret sonograms and to help them learn to see (Sandelowski 1994b, Mitchell 2001). The case of 4D 'bonding scans' provides a new context in which to explore these issues. I have argued that scanning for bonding is also a 'hybrid practice' (Taylor 1998), but one in which the priorities are reversed and the social meanings of ultrasound take precedence. Nonetheless, the sonographer must adopt an expert role to confirm the health of the fetus, sex the baby, offer reassurance and help clients to get their bearings and learn to see the fetus on the screen.

Despite the clarity and realism of 3/4D scan imagery, it is not always easily legible to the untrained eye. Observations of ultrasound scanning contrast with the typical public 3D images that are widely reproduced in the media. While the iconic, 'technofetus' is represented head up, centre frame in a clear, portrait-like image, the real-time images can be quite different. With no time for editing or manipulating the image, the picture is often indistinct. The position of the fetus, the placenta and the umbilical cord all affect the quality of the image and it can be difficult to catch a glimpse of an 'uncooperative' fetus. My observations reveal the emotional and discursive work that goes into making ultrasound imagery meaningful. Even 4D sonograms cannot be read easily or without ambiguity but are open to multiple 'codings' that reflect the circumstances of image production, image consumption and family life. Despite the greater clarity of 3/4D ultrasound for a lay audience, the images produced are not fixed; rather their meaning is fluid and multiple.

As clients grow in confidence, they take an active role in narrating the images on the screen. While the sonographer can translate the image on the screen into a signifier of a baby, women and their companions have the necessary family knowledge to construct the sonogram as a signifier of their baby, and to begin to weave the baby into a kinship network through narratives of family resemblance in appearance, personality and behaviour. Here I have described collaboration between clients and sonographers.

The 'collaborative coding' of scans reported here is remarkably similar to that described by Mitchell (2001) in her ethnography of clinical, 2D antenatal ultrasound in Canada. This continuity suggests that the cultural norms and conventions of interacting with ultrasound imagery have evolved over time and persist through technological development. Similar cultural scripts are mobilised by women and families interacting with 3/4D compared to 2D ultrasound. However, I have proposed some points of difference.

The latest 3/4D ultrasound shows the fetus with remarkable realism and makes new details available to both medical and lay viewers. Surface rendering and 3/4D technology makes facial appearance and movements or 'expressions' newly visible. While this has some clinical application (such as examining suspected facial clefts in detail), it has also been claimed by some campaigners as evidence of fetal personhood and consciousness (Palmer 2009a). In the context of bonding scans, imagery of facial appearance and 'expressions' become previously unavailable resources for narrative construction and storytelling. Bonding scan clients draw on the imagery on the screen as a means of producing personalised narratives that draw on family knowledge and familiarity to make kinship connections of resemblance and character between the soon-to-be-baby and expectant parents, and that inform imagined interactions. While commentary on family resemblance is not new, 3/4D images provide more legible images within which to note family traits. Fetal personality has commonly been inferred from ultrasound images, according to Mitchell (2001) and others, but real-time, moving, imagery of facial 'expressions' including smiles, frowns, and yawns are specific to 4D ultrasound. This new repertoire of images lends itself to elaborate narratives of fetal personality. They are also a source of great viewing pleasure and facilitate a reading of the pictures on the screen as a newborn baby. Expectant parents delight in seeing a smiling, laughing baby or even a serious-faced or grumpy baby and in enacting an imagined interaction with the soon-to-be-baby.

The observations presented here suggest that 3/4D 'bonding scans' both distance the fetus from the female body and give women an opportunity to convey their embodied experiences differently to partners and family members. As Sandelowski (1994b) has described, ultrasound has the capacity to dislocate the fetus from the pregnant subject, displaying it on the screen in such a way as to equalise the relationship of all viewers with the fetus and disrupt the special relationship pregnant woman have with their fetuses. The process of 'collaborative coding' presented here does not necessarily favour the interpretations of women but produces a narrative through cooperation between women, their partners, any other family members present, and sonographers. Commercial bonding scans give an opportunity for as many family members to be present as the client chooses (whereas hospitals tend to limit appointments to just women and their partners) and therefore, it is possible to observe a process of narrating the screen that involves more people, and people with different relationships with the soon-to-be-baby than previously described in the literature. The distinctions between roles for different family members in the scan room warrants further research and analysis.

While the study presented here partly supports Sandelowski's (1994b) contention that ultrasound equalises observers' relationship to the fetus, it also suggests that women lay claim to the images on the screen to explain their somatic experiences of pregnancy, both to themselves and to others. The position of the fetus as shown on the screen can, for example, convey the reason for physical discomfort. Women may say to their male partners, 'See! You have to believe me now when I say that she is kicking me!' Rather than being disembodied spectators, women actively relate the images on the screen to their embodied experiences of pregnancy and encourage their partners to also make links between the two.

We might wonder whether the ease with which women feel able to interpret 3/4D scan images and relate the image to their own body paves the way for a shift of power in terms of who interprets the images. Once they have their bearings, expectant parents may feel empowered to narrate the imagery, with minimal expert help needed. The explicit focus of commercial scanning on bonding, reassurance, and getting 'baby's first picture', rather than diagnostics, might also enable pregnant women and their families to impose their own interpretations on the images. In this scan room, social meanings take priority. Both sonographers and expectant parents possess expertise in interpreting the pictures in a way that is socially and personally meaningful. Indeed, intimate knowledge of family appearance, personality, and behaviour is necessary to code the sonogram not just as 'a baby', but 'our baby'. Finally, in this case, women and their families have more control over the function of ultrasound in their pregnancy and social lives. They elect to attend such scans for their own reasons. However, more research is needed to understand the reasons for choosing 'bonding scans' and to understand how women and their families experience them. Further insight might be achieved in the future through interviews with pregnant women, their families and sonographers.

Acknowledgements

My thanks to the women and their families who allowed me to observe their scans. Thanks also to the sonographers who took part in the study. I am grateful for the support of Dr. Ann Kaloski who supervised the fieldwork presented here. This article is based on my doctoral research undertaken at the Centre for Women's Studies, University of York and funded by the Arts and Humanities Research Council (AHRC). Please note that this research was undertaken using my previous name of Julie Palmer.

References

Beech, B. (2005) Ultrasound *AIMS* 17(1). Available at: http://www.aims.org.uk/Journal/Vol17No1/ultrasound.htm. Date last accessed 28 March 2006.

Berlant, L. (1994) America, "fat", the fetus, *Boundary* 2, 21, 145–95.

Brezinka, C. (2010) Nonmedical use of ultrasound in pregnancy: ethical issues, patients' rights and potential misuse, *Ultrasound in Medicine & Biology*, 36, 8, 1233–6.

Bricker, L., Garcia, J., Henderson, J., Mugford, M., Neilson, J., Roberts, T. and Martin, M.-A. (2000) Ultrasound screening in pregnancy: a systematic review of the clinical effectiveness, cost effectiveness and women's views, *Health Technology Assessment*, 4, 1, 1–193.

British Medical Ultrasound Society (2007) *ECMUS statement on souvenir scanning approved and endorsed by BMUS Council*. Available at: http://www.bmus.org/policies-guides/pg-safety05.asp. Date last accessed 29 September 2010.

Casper, M.J. (1998) *The Making of the Unborn Patient: A Social Anatomy of Fetal Surgery*. New Brunswick, NJ: Rutgers University Press.

Chervenak, F.A. (2005) An ethical critique of boutique fetal imaging: a case for the medicalization of fetal imaging, *American Journal of Obstetrics and Gynaecology*, 192, 1, 31–3.

Clement, S., Wilson, J. and Sikorski, J. (1998) Women's experiences of antenatal ultrasound scans. In Clement, S. (ed) *Psychological Perspectives on Pregnancy and Childbirth*. Edinburgh: Churchill Livingstone.

Chrysanthou, M. (2002) Transparency and selfhood: utopia and the informed body, *Social Science & Medicine*, 54, 3, 469–79.

Draper, J. (2002) 'It was a real good show': the ultrasound scan, fathers and the power of visual knowledge, *Sociology of Health & Illness*, 24, 6, 771–95.

Duden, B. (1993) *Disembodying Women: Perspectives on Pregnancy & the Unborn*. Cambridge, MA: Harvard University Press.

Franklin, S. (1991) Fetal fascinations: new dimensions of the medical-scientific construction of fetal personhood. In Lury, C. and Stacey, J. (eds) *Off-centre: Feminism and Cultural Studies*. London: HarperCollins Academic.

Gammeltoft, T. and Nguyên, H.T.T. (2007) The commodification of obstetric ultrasound scanning in Hanoi, Viet Nam, *Reproductive Health Matters*, 15, 2, 163–71.

Garcia, J., Bricker, L., Henderson, J., Martin, M.-A., Mugford, M., Nielson, J., *et al.* (2002) Women's views of pregnancy ultrasound: a systematic review, *Birth*, 29, 4, 225–50.

Gudex, C., Nielsen, B.L. and Madsen, M. (2006) Why women want prenatal ultrasound in normal pregnancy, *Ultrasound in Obstetrics & Gynecology*, 27, 2, 145–50.

Gunderman, R.B. (2005) The medical community's changing vision of the patient: the importance of radiology, *Radiology*, 234, 2, 339–42.

Health Protection Agency (2010) Advisory group on non-ionising radiation (AGNIR). Available at: http://www.hpa.org.uk/Topics/Radiation/RadiationAdvisoryGroups/AdvisoryGroupOnNonIonisingRadiation. Date accessed 29 September 2010.

Henwood, F. (2001) In/different screening: contesting medical knowledge in an antenatal setting. In Henwood, F., Kennedy, H. and Miller, N. (eds) *Cyborg Lives? Women's Technobiographies*. York: Raw Nerve.

ISUOG Bioeffects and Safety Committee, Abramowicz, J.S., Kossoff, G., Marsal, K. and Ter Haar, G. & On Behalf of the Executive Board of the International Society for Ultrasound in Obstetrics and Gynaecology (2002) Safety statement 2000 (reconfirmed 2002), *Ultrasound in Obstetrics and Gynaecology*, 19, 1, 105.

Kroløkke, C. (2010) On a trip to the womb: biotourist metaphors in fetal ultrasound imaging, *Women's Studies in Communication*, 33, 2, 138–53.

Kurjak, A., Miskovic, B., Andonotopo, W., Azumendi, G. and Vrcic, H. (2007) How useful is 3D and 4D ultrasound in perinatal medicine? *Journal of Perinatal Medicine*, 35, 1, 10–27.

Lee, H.R. and Paterson, A.M. (2004) Sonographers and registration to practice, *Ultrasound*, 12, 1, 64–7.

Mehaffy, M.M. (2000) Fetal attractions: the limit of cyborg theory, *Women's Studies*, 29, 2, 177–94.

Mitchell, L.M. (2001) *Baby's First Picture: Ultrasound and the Politics of Fetal Subjects*. Toronto: University of Toronto Press.

Mitchell, L.M. and Georges, E. (1997) Cross-cultural cyborgs: Greek and Canadian discourses on fetal ultrasound, *Feminist Studies*, 23, 2, 373–401.

National Collaborating Centre for Women's and Children's Health (2003) *Antenatal Care: Routine Care for the Healthy Pregnant Woman.* London: NICE.

Oakley, A. (1984) *The Captured Womb: A History of the Medical Care of Pregnant Women.* Oxford: Basil Blackwell Publisher Ltd.

Ockleford, E., Berryman, J. and Hsu, R. (2003) Do women understand prenatal screening for fetal abnormality? *British Journal of Midwifery*, 11, 7, 445–9.

Palmer, J. (2007) *The visible techno-foetus: ultrasound imagery and its non-medical significances in everyday contexts.* PhD. University of York.

Palmer, J. (2009a) Seeing and knowing: ultrasound images in the contemporary abortion debate, *Feminist Theory*, 10, 2, 173–89.

Palmer, J. (2009b) The placental body in 4D: everyday practices of non-diagnostic sonography, *Feminist Review*, 93, 1, 64–80.

Petchesky, R.P. (1987) Fetal images: the power of visual culture in the politics of reproduction. In Stanworth, M. (ed) *Reproductive Technologies: Gender, Motherhood and Medicine.* Cambridge and Oxford: Polity Press in association with Basil Blackwell.

Sandelowski, M. (1994a) Channel of desire: fetal ultrasonography in two use-contexts, *Qualitative Health Research*, 4, 3, 262–80.

Sandelowski, M. (1994b) Separate, but less unequal: fetal ultrasonography and the transformation of expectant mother/fatherhood, *Gender and Society*, 8, 2, 230–45.

Smith, R.P., Titmarsh, S. and Overton, T.G. (2004) Improving patients' knowledge of the fetal anomaly scan. *Ultrasound in Obstetrics and Gynaecology*, 24, 7, 740–4.

The Society and College of Radiographers (2009) Developing and growing the sonographer workforce: education and training needs. Available at: http://www.sor.org/public/document-library/sor_ultrasound_workforce_development.pdf. Date last accessed 13 October 2010.

Stabile, C.A. (1994) *Feminism and the Technological Fix.* Manchester: Manchester University Press.

Tanne, J.H. (2004) FDA warns against commercial prenatal ultrasound videos, *British Medical Journal*, 328, 7444, 853.

Taylor, J.S. (1998) Image of contradiction: obstetrical ultrasound in American culture. In Franklin, S. and Ragoné, H. (eds) *Reproducing Reproduction: Kinship, Power and Technological Innovation.*, Philadelphia, PA: University of Pennsylvania Press.

Taylor, J.S. (2008) *The Public Life of the Fetal Sonogram: Technology, Consumption and the Politics of Reproduction.* New Brunswick, NJ: Rutgers University Press.

Thorpe, K., Harker, L., Pike, A. and Marlow, N. (1993) Women's views of ultrasonography: a comparison of women's experiences of antenatal ultrasound screening with cerebral ultrasound of their newborn infant, *Social Science & Medicine*, 36, 3, 311–15.

van Dijck, J. (2005) *The Transparent Body: A Cultural Analysis of Medical Imaging.* Seattle, WA: University of Washington Press.

Voelker, R. (2005) The business of baby pictures: controversy brews over "keepsake" fetal ultrasounds, *Journal of American Medical Association*, 293, 1, 25–7.

Watts, G. (2007) First pictures: one for the album, *British Medical Journal*, 334, 7587, 232–33.

Index

abortion 136
ageing 37
ambient risk 33
amniocentesis 106, 111, 112, 113, 114, 115, 116, 125
animal experiments 129
anomalous findings 50–51, 57
antenatal screening 11–12
  amniocentesis 106, 111, 112, 113, 114, 115, 116, 125
  choice 105, 121, 122
  conflict 116
  conversation analytic studies 105, 106
  decision-making 105, 106, 121, 123
  Denmark 122
  Down's syndrome 108, 109, 110, 116, 117
  first trimester prenatal risk assessment
    (FTPRA) 122–9
  high-risk results 106, 108, 114
  Hong Kong 107, 108, 109, 117
  knowledge production 123, 132, 133
    resistance 128–30
  non-directiveness 106, 112, 121, 122, 123, 130–131,
    132
  presumed acceptance 106
  social characteristics of patients 4, 5, 11, 107, 109,
    115, 117, 118
  ultrasound scans 116, 124–7
    bonding scans 11, 12, 136, 138–40, 142, 146, 147
    collaborative coding 142–6, 147
    communicating risk with care 127–31, 132
    feminist critiques 136, 137, 139–40, 142, 145
    fetal facial expressions 140, 144, 147
    fetal personality 143–4
    fetal resemblance 142–3
    medical and social meanings 137–8, 146, 148
    potential harm 138, 139
    sonographer as expert guide 141–2, 146–7
    sonographers' body language 127
    speaking to and for the fetus 144–5
    technological and embodied knowledge 145–6,
      147, 148
armed forces 19–20, 27
attendance 6
  see also non-attendance
autonomous decision-making 28, 29, 122, 132

blood pressure 25
blood tests 35
Blume, S. 76

bonding scans 11, 12, 136, 138–40, 142, 146, 147
breast screening 3, 4, 26, 28
bridging work 9, 10, 48, 52, 53, 56–7

cancer screening 21, 60
  cervical see cervical screening; HPV
  prostate see prostate cancer detection; prostate-
    specific antigen tests
cardiovascular disease 20, 22, 23
case finding 27–8
cervical screening 4, 5–6, 10, 21
  diagnostics companies 73
    see also Digene
  molecularisation 73, 79, 84, 86
  Pap smear 73, 74–5, 79, 84, 86
  see also HPV
choice 105, 121, 122
  see also autonomous decision-making; informed
    choice
cholesterol 34–5, 36, 37, 38, 39, 40–41, 42
chronic illness 21–2, 42
citizenship 7, 68
coercion 122
commercial markets 74, 75, 85
communicable diseases 19, 20, 27
communication 127–31, 132
conversation analysis 11, 105, 106
corporatisation 74, 75, 85
costs of screening 2, 3

decision-making 6–7, 11, 105, 106, 121, 123
Denmark 122
Despret, Vinciane 129, 131
diabetes 20
diagnosis 2, 50
diagnostics companies 10, 73, 74
  see also Digene
Digene 73, 74, 75
  collaboration with Kaiser Permanenete 79, 81
  HC2 test 79–80, 81
  Hybrid Capture test 75, 78
  protecting market share 82–4
  strategic success 84, 85–6
DNA patenting 73, 74
Down's syndrome 108, 109, 110, 116, 117

embodiment 6, 38, 145–6, 147, 148
epidemiology 94

The Sociology of Medical Screening, First Edition. Edited by Natalie Armstrong and Helen Eborall.
Chapters © 2012 The Authors. Book Compilation © 2012 Foundation for the Sociology of Health
& Illness / Blackwell Publishing Ltd. Published 2012 by Blackwell Publishing Ltd.